Pharmacokinetics

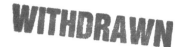

Pharmacokinetics

Processes and Mathematics

Peter G. Welling

ACS Monograph 185

American Chemical Society
Washington, DC   1986

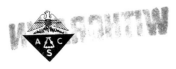

Library of Congress Cataloging-in-Publication Data

Welling, Peter G.
   Pharmacokinetics.
   (ACS monograph; 185)

   Bibliography: p.
   Includes index.

   1. Pharmacokinetics.

   I. Title. II. Series.

RM301.5.W45   1986   615'.7   86-20644
ISBN 0-8412-0967-7

To Graham, Christine, and Stephen

FOREWORD

ACS MONOGRAPH SERIES was started by arrangement with the interallied Conference of Pure and Applied Chemistry, which met in London and Brussels in July 1919, when the American Chemical Society undertook the production and publication of Scientific and Technological Monographs on chemical subjects. At the same time it was agreed that the National Research Council, in cooperation with the American Chemical Society and the American Physical Society, should undertake the production and publication of Critical Tables of Chemical and Physical Constants. The American Chemical Society and the National Research Council mutually agreed to care for these two fields of chemical progress.

The Council of the American Chemical Society, acting through its Committee on National Policy, appointed editors and associates to select authors of competent authority in their respective fields and to consider critically the manuscripts submitted. The first Monograph appeared in 1921. Since 1944 the Scientific and Technological Monographs have been combined in the Series.

These Monographs are intended to serve two principal purposes: first, to make available to chemists a thorough treatment of a selected area in a form usable by persons working in more or less unrelated fields so that they may correlate their own work with a larger area of physical science; and second, to stimulate further research in the specific field treated. To implement this purpose, the authors of Monographs give extended references to the literature.

ABOUT THE AUTHOR

PETER G. WELLING, a native of London, obtained his B.Sc., M.Sc., and Ph.D. degrees from Sydney University in Australia. After completing postdoctoral studies at the University of Michigan and a brief period at Pfizer (U.K.), he joined the faculty of the School of Pharmacy at the University of Wisconsin in 1978. In 1984, he joined Warner-Lambert/Parke-Davis as Director of the Department of Pharmacokinetics and Drug Metabolism.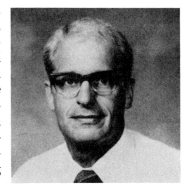

Dr. Welling has published over 150 research articles and reviews, and two books on pharmacokinetics. He served as permanent member on the Pharmacology Study Section at the National Institutes of Health, and is an editor of *Antimicrobial Agents and Chemotherapy*. He was awarded the D.Sc. degree from Sydney University in 1980.

CONTENTS

THE MATHEMATICS OF PHARMACOKINETICS

PREFACE

THE STUDY OF PHARMACOKINETICS was first formalized in 1937 by Torsten Teorell. After that time, interest in the subject grew steadily, and in the 1960s pharmacokinetics as a discipline underwent considerable expansion. Those concerned with drug discovery and development realized the importance of pharmacokinetics, and the study of pharmacokinetics was made more accurate and easier by two developments: sophisticated analytical procedures capable of measuring small concentrations of substances in biological fluids, and computers and computer software.

During my years at the University of Wisconsin, I taught courses in basic, clinical, and advanced pharmacokinetics. During the preparation and teaching of these courses, I was repeatedly reminded of the need for a basic understanding of physical pharmacy, physiology, anatomy, and pathology in order to comprehend and practice pharmacokinetic principles. Without this background, pharmacokinetics becomes a mathematical "black box" and cannot be used effectively.

The purpose of this book is to address this need. The first part of the book is devoted to the processes involved in drug absorption, distribution, metabolism, excretion, membrane transport, and the various factors influencing these phenomena. The second part of the book is devoted to the mathematics of pharmacokinetics. The student is invited to read the two parts sequentially because many of the mathematical treatments are predicated on concepts described in earlier chapters. The pharmacokinetic topics are presented in order of increasing complexity, from the relatively simple one-compartment kinetic model to multicompartment and physiological models and nonlinear kinetics.

Each chapter contains a list of cited literature, which also serves as a reading list to guide the reader to selected key publications. Many of the chapters also have solved problems. These are included because I am convinced that the only way to grasp the concepts of pharmacokinetics is to use them repeatedly.

I am indebted to G. L. Amidon, P. Corrick-West, and A. Selen for their help in developing the original courses during early and more recent times, and also to John Wagner and Adrian Ryan for introducing me to this business. I am indebted to Donna Burrows for her painstaking typing of the manuscript. Lastly, I wish to thank my family for putting up with it all.

PETER G. WELLING

Pharmaceutical Research Division
Warner-Lambert/Parke-Davis
Ann Arbor, MI 48105

DRUG ABSORPTION, DISTRIBUTION, METABOLISM, AND EXCRETION

1

Introduction

Definitions

Pharmacokinetics is a relatively new discipline and, as the name implies, it is the study of the rate of change of drug concentrations in the body. Pharmacokinetics is not to be confused with the closely related subject pharmacodynamics, which is concerned with the time relationships of the pharmacological response elicited by a drug. A third related subject, pharmacology, is the study of the change in organ function elicited by a drug.

Separating these three processes is not really possible when observing the action of a drug in the body. Each process plays an important role, and the final observed response to an administered drug is a complex function of all three.

Although the pharmacokinetic behavior of a particular compound may be complex, the mathematics associated with pharmacokinetic processes is quite fundamental. The description of even the most complex pharmacokinetic behavior can be readily understood if one appreciates the "building block" nature of pharmacokinetic modeling.

Background

Before the many complex relationships involved in pharmacokinetic processes were understood, drugs were administered purely on an empirical basis. What happened to a drug after it entered the body, or how its fate might influence the therapeutic effect, was not appreciated. The birth of

0065-7719/86/0185-0003$06.00/1

modern pharmacokinetics occurred in 1937 with the publication of two classic papers by the Swedish scientist, Torsten Teorell (1,2). The papers give the basic equations for drug absorption, distribution, and elimination following various types of administration.

The next major resurgence of interest in pharmacokinetics, and one that continues to this day, occurred in the late 1950s and early 1960s. During this period, tremendous advances were made in this area of research. Today, pharmacokinetic concepts are used at all stages of drug discovery, development, and therapy. For example, all new drug submissions to regulatory agencies must now include pharmacokinetic information; efficacy and toxicity studies are no longer valid unless blood level or urinary excretion data are obtained simultaneously. Also, pharmacokinetic principles are being used routinely in the design and optimization of drug formulations and dosage regimens.

Different Approaches of Pharmacokinetics

Pharmacokinetics has tended to diverge into three major philosophical approaches: compartment modeling, physiological modeling, and model-independent pharmacokinetics.

In the compartment modeling approach, the body is assumed to be made up of one or more compartments. These compartments may be spacial or chemical in nature. For example, if a drug is converted in the body to a metabolite, then the metabolite may be considered a separate compartment to the parent drug. In most cases, however, the compartment is used to represent a body volume or group of similar tissues or fluids into which a drug distributes. Typical compartment models of this type are illustrated in Figure 1.1.

In the physiological model approach, pharmacokinetic interpretation is based on known anatomical or physiological values. Unlike the compartment modeling approach, in which drug movement between compartments is based largely on reversible or irreversible first-order processes, drug movement using the physiological model approach is based on blood flow rates through particular organs or tissues and experimentally determined blood–tissue concentration ratios. The basic unit that describes the relationship between blood and a particular target tissue is shown in Figure 1.2, and a typical physiological model is shown in Figure 1.3.

The main advantages of the physiological model are that drug movement can be predicted in specific organs and tissues, and that changes in tissue perfusion due to pathological conditions, such as fever or congestive heart failure, can be taken into account when predicting tissue levels. The main disadvantage of the physiological model is that the associated mathematics can become complex and unwieldy. Models must also be

ONE-COMPARTMENT OPEN MODEL, BOLUS INTRAVENOUS INJECTION

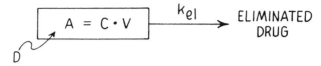

TWO-COMPARTMENT OPEN MODEL, ORAL ADMINISTRATION

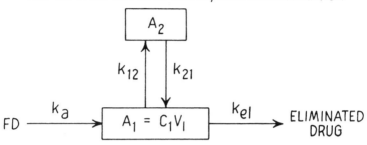

Figure 1.1. Typical compartment models. One-compartment: D is the dose, A is the amount of drug in the body, C is the concentration of drug in distribution volume V, and k_{el} is the first-order rate constant for drug elmination. Two-compartment: FD is fraction of dose absorbed, k_{12} and k_{21} first-order rate constants for transfer of drug between compartments, and k_a is the first-order rate constant for drug absorption. Subscripts denote first (central) or second (peripheral) compartments.

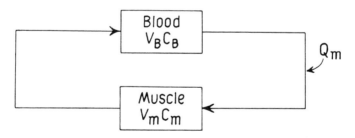

Figure 1.2. Basic physiological model unit. Q_m is the blood flow rate through organ, V is the organ volume, C is the drug concentration. Subscript denotes the organ, in this case blood (B) or muscle (m).

developed in vitro or in experimental animals because it is difficult or impossible to validate a model in humans. The physiological model approach has been used extensively for anticancer compounds and for other agents where drug or metabolite location at particular tissues or organs is important.

Model-independent pharmacokinetics represents a recent trend away from complex modeling systems toward a less complex approach based

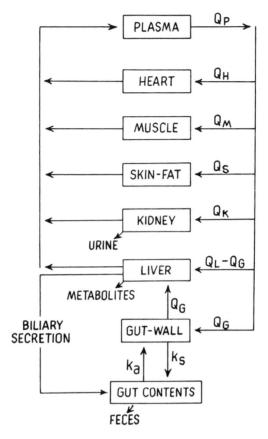

Figure 1.3. Complete physiological model for digoxin disposition in the rat. (Reproduced with permission from J. Pharm. Sci., **1977,** 66, 1138).

purely on mathematical description of blood or plasma profiles of drug or metabolites, and calculation of useful pharmacokinetic values without invoking a particular model. The essence of this approach to pharmacokinetics is that it avoids the use of kinetic parameters that cannot readily be validated, and kinetic parameters that have little anatomical or physiological significance. This approach is useful in situations where kinetic parameters such as absorption and elimination rates and clearances are required, but specific distribution characteristics are less important.

Literature Cited

1. Teorell, T. *Arch. Int. Pharmacodyn.* **1937,** 57, 205–225.
2. Teorell, T. *Arch. Int. Pharmacodyn.* **1937,** 57, 226–240.

2

Parenteral Routes of Drug Administration

Some drugs are used for topical or local effects, for example, local anesthetics, topical antibacterial agents, fungicides, or drugs used in the eye. Other drugs have to be absorbed into the systemic circulation or blood stream to exert their therapeutic effect. The latter group, called *systemically acting drugs,* is of interest to us. These drugs may be administered by routes that fall into two major categories: enteral and parenteral. *Enteral* administration applies to drugs administered via the gastrointestinal (GI) system, and *parenteral* administration applies to drugs given by any other route. However, this definition becomes obscure in some cases.

The routes of drug administration that fall into the parenteral category are as follows:

- intravenous
- intramuscular
- subcutaneous
- intradermal
- percutaneous
- inhalation
- intraarterial
- intrathecal
- vaginal

The simplicity and good patient acceptance of the oral dosing route are such that parenteral routes are generally used only when the oral route

0065-7719/86/0185-0007$06.00/1

is inappropriate, for example, with drugs that are unstable in the GI tract or are poorly absorbed after oral doses. Parenteral routes may also be used when prompt onset of action is required or when a patient simply cannot take oral medication.

Intravenous and Intramuscular Administration

Intravenous administration is the method used to introduce drug directly into the venous circulation by means of a syringe or an intravenous line. This method results in complete absorption of drug or complete bio-availability, but the shape of the resulting drug profile in plasma is determined by the rate of injection as indicated in Figure 2.1. The complete systemic availability of drugs given by this route makes it extremely useful when investigating the absorption efficiency or absolute bioavailability of drugs administered by other routes. In fact, regulatory agencies prefer intravenous doses to be used whenever possible for this purpose in drug absorption studies.

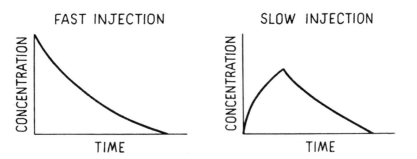

Figure 2.1. *Profiles of drug concentration versus time in blood after fast and slow intravenous injection.*

The intravenous bolus route is particularly useful when a prompt effect is required (1). A good example of this method of administration is the use of intravenous lidocaine in emergency treatment of cardiac arrhythmia. A major disadvantage of the intravenous route is that once injected, the dose cannot be withdrawn. Therefore, it is common practice to inject the drug slowly over a period of several minutes to avoid excessively high initial drug levels. Precise and continuous drug therapy is obtained by constant intravenous infusion, which is generally achieved by intravenous drip or infusion pump.

Intramuscular injection may be used for drugs that are not absorbed orally but for which rapid drug levels in the blood, such as those obtained after bolus intravenous doses, are not necessary (1). Drugs given by intramuscular injection include the aminoglycosides, some cephalosporins, and penicillins. Most but not all compounds are rapidly and reliably absorbed from intramuscular doses. Slow or incomplete absorption from intramuscular sites has been reported for chlordiazepoxide, diazepam, digoxin, phenytoin, phenobarbital, and promethazine. A number of factors may be responsible for incomplete absorption from intramuscular injections. These factors include degradation of drug in the muscle tissue and slow absorption of some injected material leading to low and possibly undetectable levels in the blood after the bulk of drug has been absorbed into the bloodstream. Drug may also precipitate at the injection site, and thus slow or poor absorption would result.

Several other factors can influence drug absorption from intramuscular injections. The type of solvent may be important. Drugs with low aqueous solubility like diazepam can be dissolved in nonaqueous vehicles such as propylene glycol and mineral oil. Drugs administered in this way may precipitate at the injection site, and imperfect absorption would result. Injection volume and molecular size may influence intramuscular drug absorption. Small injection volumes generally lead to faster absorption than large volumes. Absorption of lipid-soluble substances is essentially independent of molecular size, and absorption of water-soluble drugs is inversely proportional to molecular size. Small water-soluble molecules readily enter the circulation via the blood capillaries at the injection site, whereas larger molecules must enter the circulatory system indirectly via the lymphatics. Vascular perfusion, which is the blood flow rate through muscular tissue, ranges from approximately 0.02 to 0.07 mL/min per gram of muscle tissue. The higher the flow rate, the faster the rate at which drug is cleared from the injection site. The absorption rate of insulin zinc in children has been shown to be faster from an arm injection than than from a thigh injection, and this increased rate may be due to the greater vascular perfusion and smaller mass of arm muscle tissue.

Because of the generally nondestructive nature of the muscular environment and the virtual absence of a time limit during which a drug dosage form can remain in that region, the intramuscular site is ideal for sustained or controlled drug release.

Sustained release from intramuscularly implanted devices has recently been reviewed by Chien (2). Approaches that have been used for sustained drug release include aqueous suspensions for such compounds as penicillin G benzathine and penicillin G procaine; oily vehicles, in which drug release is controlled by partitioning between the vehicle and the surrounding aqueous medium; and complex formation, in which drug is complexed with materials such as methylcellulose and slowly released.

Two other methods that are being actively investigated to obtain sustained drug release from intramuscular injections are polymer matrix suspensions using biodegradable polymers such as polylactic acid, and microencapsulation. Microencapsulation has recently been shown to produce prolonged release of fluphenazine embonate and other compounds, and thereby cause a twofold increase in duration of activity.

Parenteral Routes Other Than Intravenous and Intramuscular

Subcutaneous, intradermal, and percutaneous administration involve drug absorption through the skin (3). The skin is generally considered to be an impermeable barrier to most substances. However, when administered in the appropriate manner, drug substances can be effectively absorbed through the skin. As indicated in Figure 2.2, three major regions in the skin cover underlying muscle tissue: the epidermis, the dermis, and the subcutaneous regions. The region that provides the major resistance to drug penetration is the stratum corneum, which is the outer horny layer of the epithelium. If this region is intact, then penetration of drug into the body via the skin and water loss in the other direction are slow. If this region is not intact, because of burns or other injuries, then permeability in both directions is increased.

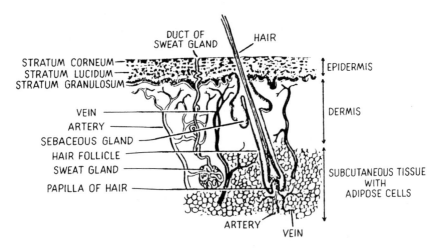

Figure 2.2. Cross section through human skin.

Drugs may penetrate the epidermis by two major routes: the transepidermal route, where compounds pass through or between the epidermal cells, and the transappendageal route, where passage occurs via the skin appendages, for example, the hair follicles or sebaceous glands. Although penetration by the transappendageal route is probably more efficient than the transepidermal route, the latter appears to be more important because of the very small percentage of skin surface made up of such structures as hair follicles (approximately 0.2%) and sweat glands (approximately 0.04%).

Subcutaneous Injection. Subcutaneous injection bypasses the epidermal and dermal skin layers and generally ensures efficient, if perhaps slow, systemic drug absorption. Many compounds are routinely given in this way, in particular insulin, local anesthetics, and vaccines. Small volumes of solutions may be given by this route, usually in the upper arm, although the anterior surface of the thigh or abdomen may also be used.

The primary absorption membrane in subcutaneous tissue is the capillary wall. This situation is similar to intramuscular injections. However, because of the lower capillary density in subcutaneous connective tissue, absorption is generally slower by this route. The absorption rate is markedly increased by rubbing or by exercise; the dramatic effect that exercise may have on insulin absorption is indicated in Figure 2.3 (4).

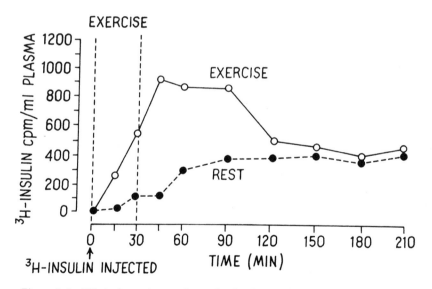

Figure 2.3. Effect of exercise on plasma levels of intact ^{3}H-insulin following subcutaneous injection of 4 × 105 cpm of ^{3}H-insulin/kg body weight into the leg of a juvenile patient. (Reproduced with permission from reference 4. Copyright 1979, American Diabetes Association.)

The site of injection is also important, as shown in Figure 2.4 (5). A much greater hypoglycemic effect was observed after injection of insulin into an exercised leg compared to the arm or abdomen.

Use of subcutaneous implants or similar techniques is another pop-

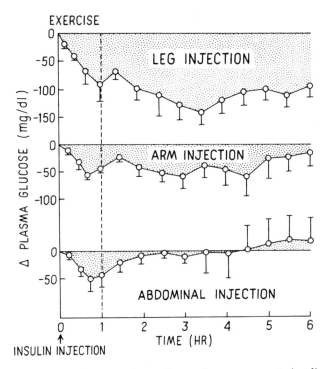

Figure 2.4. *Influence of injection site on plasma glucose response to insulin during leg exercise. Shaded areas represent changes in plasma glucose levels (mean ± SE) following insulin injection during leg exercise compared to plasma glucose levels obtained with no exercise. The area above the curve for leg injection is significantly greater than those for both arm (p < 0.02) and abdominal (p < 0.005) injections. (Reproduced with permission from reference 5. Copyright 1978, Massachusetts Medical Society.)*

ular and expanding area for sustained-release medication, and commercial implants are available for certain steroid hormones, penicillin, gold salts, and sulfonamides. Other commercial implants are being actively investigated.

Intradermal Injection. Unlike subcutaneous injections, intradermal injections are usually intended for local effect. However, this route also has potential for systemic activity, particularly for vaccines. In one study, an intradermal injection of 0.1 mL of an Asian influenza vaccine produced an effect comparable to that of a 1-mL subcutaneous injection of the same vaccine (6).The intradermal route thus may not only cause less local irritation compared to the subcutaneous route, but may also be particularly useful in situations of vaccine shortage because of the smaller dosage volumes required for a given effect.

Percutaneous Absorption. Percutaneous absorption occurs after topical administration of drug to the skin surface. In this situation, the drug has to cross the entire thickness of the skin, including the stratum corneum, before it can enter the systemic circulation. Therefore, percutaneous absorption may be considered an unlikely route for most compounds. However, in certain cases, if the compound is retained on the skin surface for a sufficiently long period of time, and if the skin surface is kept in a sufficiently hydrated condition, percutaneous absorption may be efficient. Percutaneous administration for systemic effect is a practical dosage route only for drugs given in small doses of 2–5 mg or less.

The concept of effective percutaneous administration has found application in the new topical or percutaneous sustained-release dosage forms of antianginal agents such as nitroglycerin. Slow absorption of drug from these formulations, due partly to slow release from the topical device, leads to low circulating drug levels that may provide prophylaxis against angina. If fast relief is required, for example, in the treatment of an angina attack, then the percutaneous route is useless and a more direct dosage route is required. For controlled drug release, however, the percutaneous route appears to have considerable potential, and much more will be heard of this route of administration during the next few years.

Inhalation. When a substance is taken by inhalation, it is presented to the membranes of the mouth or nose, the pharynx, trachea, bronchi, bronchioles, alveolar sacs, and alveoli (7). Together, these regions, illustrated in Figure 2.5, constitute an extremely large surface area for rapid absorption that occurs mostly in the alveolar ducts, alveolar sacs, and alveoli. Drugs may be introduced into the respiratory system as gases or as inhalation aerosols. Examples of the former are general anesthetics such as ether or chloroform. Diffusion across the alveolar–capillary membrane offers no significant resistance to gas transfer between lung and blood, and absorption is almost instantaneous.

The active ingredient in aerosols is usually dissolved or suspended in a liquid propellant system. Upon inhalation, the aerosol contents may be deposited in regions of the respiratory tree representing different levels of penetration by impaction, sedimentation, or diffusion. Impaction generally occurs in the nasopharynx and the tracheobronchial tree when the air stream carrying the particles changes direction. Aerosol particles larger than 10 μm are deposited mostly in the nasopharyngeal region, and smaller particles penetrate more deeply into the respiratory tree.

Sedimentation rate is governed by Stokes' law and is therefore related to particle density and to the square of the particle radius. Thus, both impaction and sedimentation tend to remove larger and more dense particles in the upper respiratory tract, and result in poor and variable absorption. Smaller particles penetrate deeper and tend to be more ef-

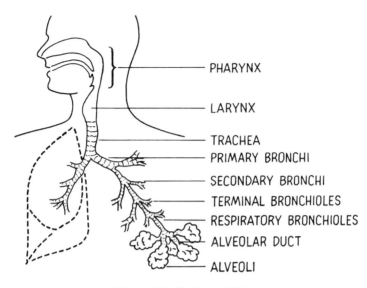

Figure 2.5. The bronchial tree.

ficiently absorbed. The relationship between regional deposition and particle size is illustrated in Table 2.1.

Inhaled aerosols are used primarily for local effect, for example, isoproterenol or metaproterenol in acute asthma attacks. They are used to a much smaller extent for systemic effects, for example, some antibiotics, atropine, and corticosteroids. One obstacle to more extensive use of this dosage route is the concern for dose accuracy. How much drug is actually inhaled and how much is swallowed? Further improvements

Table 2.1—Regional Distribution of Unit Density Spheres in Relation to Particle Size

Particle Diameter (μm)	Nasopharyngeal Region	Tracheobronchial Region	Pulmonary Region	Total
0.01	0	31	51	82
0.06	0	7	59	66
0.20	0	3	28	31
0.60	0	2	20	22
1.0	4	3	25	32
2.0	41	5	35	81
3.0	55	7	31	93
4.0	65	8	24	97
6.0	80	9	10	99
10.0	99	0.7	0.2	100

NOTE: All results are percent aerosol deposition for tidal volume of 750 mL.
SOURCE: Reproduced with permission from reference 7. Copyright 1973, Lea & Febiger.

of inhalation devices will expand the use of this highly efficient method of drug administration.

Intraarterial Administration. Intraarterial injection or infusion is used predominantly for regional delivery of drugs to specific organs or tissues, for example, in cancer chemotherapy or in the use of vasopressin for GI bleeding. Intraarterial injection increases drug delivery to the area supplied by the infused artery while reducing access of drug, at least initially, to the systemic circulation. The ability of this technique to initially achieve a high drug level in the target area is not disputed. However, to substantially reduce the entry of potentially toxic drug to the systemic circulation, some drug must be lost by metabolism, excretion, or by chemical degradation during its passage through the target organ.

Intraarterial administration is limited by its potential dangers. Complications such as embolization, arterial occlusion, and local drug toxicity are common. Maximum care is necessary when using this route of drug administration.

Intrathecal Administration. Intrathecal, meaning literally "within the sheath," derives from the Greek word *thekes* meaning a box or sheath. Intrathecal administration is the term used when a drug is injected directly into the cerebrospinal fluid within the subarachnoid space. This route of administration ensures complete bioavailability to the central nervous system and is useful for drugs that might otherwise have difficulty crossing the blood–brain barrier. Intrathecal administration is therefore used for the treatment of serious central nervous system infections such as meningitis or ventriculitis. Intrathecal injection is also used to produce spinal anesthesia to relieve chronic pain with agents such as mepivacaine hydrochloride and prilocaine hydrochloride (8). During recent years, intrathecal chemotheraphy has gained importance for the treatment of brain tumors.

Intrathecally administered drugs are generally injected directly into the lumbar spinal subarachnoid space (lumbar puncture) or into the ventricles, frequently by means of an implanted reservoir (9). The site of injection can markedly affect penetration of drug into different regions of the central nervous system. This effect is clearly demonstrated for methotrexate in Table 2.2 (10). Intraventricular administration to monkeys led to significantly higher drug levels in whole brain tissue and in the cervical and thoracic spinal cord at 2 h. But lower drug levels were found in the lower spinal cord compared to those obtained from a lumbar spinal catheter. In fact, drug concentrations in whole brain differed almost by a factor of 30 between the two dosage routes for intrathecally administered drugs. Even after 4 h had elapsed, brain levels of drug from intraventricular dosages were almost 12 times greater than those obtained from the spinal catheter. These profound differences in distribution from

Table 2.2—Mean Levels of ³H-Methotrexate in Whole Brain and Spinal Cord Regions after Intraventricular and Intrathecal Spinal Catheter Administration to Monkeys

Tissue	2 h Postinjection			4 h Postinjection		
	IVA[a]	SC[b]	IVA/SC Ratio	IVA	SC	IVA/SC Ratio
Whole brain	4.32	0.15	28.8	8.67	0.74	11.7
Cervical spinal cord	8.46	0.86	9.8	7.13	26.1	0.3
Thoracic spinal cord	7.92	1.36	5.8	4.29	60.2	0.1
Lumbar spinal cord	5.64	9.57	0.6	1.96	121.2	0.02

NOTE: Units are micrograms per gram of tissue.
[a]Intraventricular administration.
[b]Spinal catheter.
SOURCE: Reproduced with permission from reference 10. Copyright 1978, *Journal of Neurosurgery*.

two dosage routes are due to the relatively slow movement and turnover of cerebrospinal fluid compared to blood or plasma, and also to the fact that drugs given by lumbar puncture must ascend the spinal subarachnoid space against the descending bulk of cerebrospinal fluid to reach higher regions. Because cerebrospinal fluid is formed at the ventricles, administration of drug to this region allows for thorough mixing and distribution throughout different regions of the central nervous system.

Because cerebrospinal fluid and blood exist as two distinct fluids in the body, and because cerebrospinal fluid has a relatively slow turnover rate, drugs injected intrathecally are initially distributed into a very small volume of approximately 140 mL. Therefore, intrathecal dosing tends to produce higher drug concentrations in central nervous system tissue with less risk of systemic toxicity than intravenous doses. This result may not be advantageous. For example, intrathecally administered methotrexate produces concentrations in cerebrospinal fluid that may be 100-fold higher than simultaneous plasma levels. However, toxic methotrexate levels in plasma may be more prolonged following intrathecal injection compared to intravenous or oral doses because of slow drug release from the central nervous system into the general circulation.

Intraperitoneal Administration. The peritoneal cavity is the part of the body that contains, in a reasonably neat "package", the viscera. The cavity is lined by a serous membrane called the peritoneum. This membrane, and probably other associated membranes, provides an efficient absorbing surface. Compounds that are introduced into the peritoneal cavity are absorbed efficiently into the circulation. In fact, peritoneal administration is a popular route for administering drugs to experimental animals for systemic activity. This method, particularly for rodents, is physically more convenient than oral dosing, and complete drug delivery is ensured. Most intraperitoneally administered drugs are absorbed into the splanchnic circulation in the same way as orally administered drugs.

For practical reasons, intraperitoneal dosage is not common in humans. However, in some cases it may be useful. For example, intraperitoneal insulin has been shown to produce plasma insulin levels that were intermediate between the high but transient levels obtained from intravenous injection, and the delayed but prolonged levels after subcutaneous injection. Intraperitoneal injection may be an attractive alternative to other dosage routes because it provides relatively fast absorption for systemic activity while avoiding the risks associated with intravascular dosing.

The intraperitoneal route has been used to administer anticancer drugs for the treatment of tumors that have extensive peritoneal involvement, such as cancer of the ovary, stomach, and colon. If the peritoneal permeability of drugs is slower than their clearance from plasma, this route may lead to substantially higher drug concentrations in the peritoneal cavity than in plasma. Drugs that belong in this category include methotrexate and fluorouracil.

An interesting and novel development based on intraperitoneal drug administration is continuous ambulatory peritoneal dialysis (CAPD) as an alternative to hemodialysis in patients with impaired renal function (11,12). CAPD patients instill dialysate into their own peritoneal cavity by means of a permanent indwelling peritoneal catheter, and remove the dialysate by simple gravity feed following a 6–8-h dwell time. Peritoneal dialysis is not as efficient at removing substances from the body as hemodialysis, but when done on a continuous basis it appears to work well, and patients do not have to use expensive hemodialysis equipment or hospital time. A disadvantage of self-administered CAPD is the frequent occurrence of peritonitis, which must be treated with antibiotic therapy. CAPD-induced peritonitis is often associated with positive blood cultures so that, apart from selecting the best antibiotic to treat the infecting organisms, it is important to achieve therapeutic antibiotic levels in the systemic circulation in addition to the peritoneal cavity where the primary infection occurs.

Thus, for peritonitis, drugs may be given orally or by intravenous or intramuscular injection. Drugs are given intravenously or intramuscularly to achieve adequate plasma levels in the hope that sufficient drug will equilibrate across the the peritoneum to achieve adequate levels in the peritoneal cavity. Alternately, drugs may be administered into the peritoneal cavity directly with fresh dialysate to obtain bactericidal levels in the peritoneal cavity in the hope that sufficient drug diffuses across the peritoneum in the other direction to produce appropriate systemic levels. The situation is complicated because any drug that is in the peritoneum at the end of a dialysis dwell time is lost because of subsequent dialysis exchange. It is likely that the studies appearing in future literature will describe not only how particular drugs should be used to treat CAPD-associated peritonitis, but also describe a great deal about drug transport across the peritoneum under normal and febrile conditions in general.

Vaginal Administration. The vaginal route is used primarily for local effects. However, recent studies have shown that vaginal administration of some drugs may provide rapid and complete systemic absorption. This observation has been applied to the development of the vaginal controlled-release contraceptive. One example of the ease with which compounds may be absorbed from this dosage route is shown in Figure 2.6 (13). This figure shows plasma levels of estrone and estradiol in a healthy 53-year-old woman following oral and vaginal doses of conjugated equine estrogens. The levels of both estradiol and estrone are much higher following the vaginal dose compared to the oral dose. Four out of five women who were studied in this experiment had similar results.

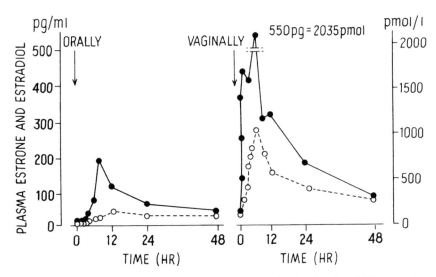

Figure 2.6. Plasma estrone (●) and estradiol (○) levels following 1.25-mg oral and vaginal doses of conjugated equine estrogens in a 53-year-old female patient. (Reproduced with permission from reference 13. Copyright 1978, British Journal of Obstetrics and Gynaecology.)

Summary

1. Parenteral routes of drug administration can be divided into those involving penetration of one or more layers of skin, for example, intradermal and percutaneous administration; those involving

penetration of serous membranes, for example, inhalation, intraperitoneal, and vaginal doses; and those involving direct targeting of drug to particular organs or regions, for example, intraarterial and intrathecal injections.

2. All parenteral dosage routes except intraperitoneal, intrathecal, and possibly intraarterial have the property that drug passes from the route of administration directly into the general circulation.

3. The fact that these drugs enter the general circulation directly is one of the major factors that differentiates parenteral from enteral dosage routes.

4. Some parenteral dosage routes, for example, intravenous, intraarterial and intrathecal injection, lead to very rapid drug availability in the body. Others, for example, percutaneous and intradermal administration, lead to slower absorption. Other parenteral dosage routes, including intramuscular and intraperitoneal injection, have intermediate properties.

5. Parenteral routes of administration are varied in nature and in their effect on drug absorption. Each method of parenteral administration has advantages and disadvantages. Advantages are related mainly to efficient absorption, accurate dosing, efficient organ targeting, absorption directly into the systemic circulation, or combinations of these. Disadvantages are related mainly to the need for sterile conditions, difficulty in retrieving a dose, inconvenience, or combinations of these. Many new approaches for drug delivery by these routes are being examined.

Literature Cited

1. Tse, F. L. S.; Welling, P. G. *J. Parenter. Drug Assoc.* **1980**, *34*, 409–421.
2. Chien, Y. W. In *Sustained and Controlled Release Drug Delivery*; Robinson, J. R., Ed.; Marcel Dekker: New York, 1978; 211–349.
3. Tse, F. L. S.; Welling, P. G. *J. Parenter. Drug Assoc.* **1980**, *34*, 484–495.
4. Berger, M.; Halban, P. A.; Assal, J. P.; Offord, R. E.; Vranic, M.; Renold, A. C. *Diabetes* **1979**, *28*, 53–57.
5. Koivisto, V. A.; Felig, P. *N. Engl. J. Med.* **1978**, *298*, 79–83.
6. Sanger, M. D. *Ann. Allergy*, **1959**, *17*, 173–178.
7. Gorman, W. G.; Dittal, G., In *Current Concepts in the Pharmaceutical Sciences: Dosage Form Design and Bioavailability*; Swarbrick, J., Ed; Lea and Febiger: Philadelphia, PA, 1973; 97–148.
8. Maher, R.; Mehta, M. In *Persistant Pain*; Lipton, S., Ed.; Academic Press: London, 1977; Vol. 1.
9. Shapiro, W. R.; Young, D. F.; Mehta, B. M. *N. Engl. J. Med.* **1975**, *293*, 161–166.
10. Yen, J.; Reiss, F. L.; Kimbelberg, H. K.; Bourke, R. S. *J. Neurosurg.* **1978**, *48*, 894–902.
11. Johnson, C. A.; Zimmerman, S. W.; Rogge, M. *Am. J. Kidney Dis.* **1984**, *4*, 3–17.
12. Rogge, M. C.; Johnson, C. A.; Zimmerman, S. W.; Welling, P. G. *Antimicrob. Ag. Chemother.* **1985**, *27*, 578–582.
13. England, D. E.; Johansson, E. D. B. *Br. J. Obstet. Gynaecol.* **1978**, *85*, 957–964.

3

Enteral Routes of Drug Administration

The enteral routes of drug administration include buccal or sublingual, gastric, intestinal, and rectal. GI absorption is by far the most common of all dosage routes, and the great majority of medicinal agents are administered this way.

The GI tract is the site of absorption for most nutrients, and it is a highly sophisticated and complex system. Therefore, it is expected that this region should be an effective absorption site for most drugs and other foreign substances. Compounds taken by the oral route are exposed to a variety of environments including wide ranges of pH; a variety of secretions such as bile, hydrochloric acid, and digestive enzymes; and different types of absorption membranes as they pass from one region of the GI tract to another (1–3). Changes in pH can affect the degree of ionization of acidic and basic drugs and can therefore influence lipophilicity. These factors can in turn influence drug absorption.

To understand how these various factors may influence drug absorption, a review of the present knowledge of membrane structure and the mechanisms of membrane transport is helpful. Much of the material discussed here applies to membranes generally and is equally important for drug distribution and elimination in addition to some types of parenteral dosing. However, most of the information available was generated from studies involving the GI tract.

0065-7719/86/0185-0021$06.00/1
© 1986 American Chemical Society

The Biological Cell Membrane

A drug must pass through one or more biological membranes to be absorbed and distributed into organs and tissues, and eventually eliminated by hepatic, renal, or other routes. Biological membranes are complex structures that serve many purposes. The GI epithelial lining is a membrane concerned with selective absorption and secretion. The membranes of the blood–brain barrier are designed to protect the brain from foreign substances, and the membranes of the proximal kidney tubules are concerned with selective drug secretion into the tubules. Some membranes are sensitive to hormonal influences. For example, the membranes associated with cells of the distal renal tubules are acted upon by vasopressin from the posterior pituitary gland, and water reabsorption results. However, the membranes of the proximal tubule cells are unaffected by vasopressin.

Despite the great diversity in membrane structure and action, a general consensus regarding the basic structure of the cell membrane exists. Opinions regarding the exact nature of the membrane continuously change as investigative methods improve. The present concept of the basic structure of the cell membrane is depicted in Figure 3.1. This model was first

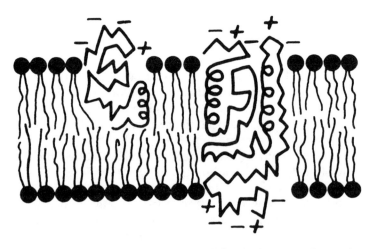

Figure 3.1.   Schematic cross-sectional view of the lipid-globular protein mosaic model of the membrane structure. The phospholipids are arranged as a discontinuous bilayer with their ionic and polar heads in contact with water. The integral proteins are shown as globular molecules partially embedded in, and partially protruding from, the membrane. The protruding parts have ionic residues (− and +) of the protein on their surfaces, and the nonpolar residues are largely in the embedded parts. Accordingly, the protein molecules are amphipathic. The degree to which the integral proteins are embedded and, in particular, whether they span the entire membrane thickness, depend on the size and structure of the molecules. (Reproduced with permission from reference 1. Copyright 1972, American Association for the Advancement of Science.).

proposed by Singer and Nicolson in 1972 (4) and represents a refinement of earlier models. The model comprises a bimolecular lipid leaflet containing phospholipids, cholesterol, and fatty acid esters that are oriented with their hydrophobic portions inside and their polar or hydrophilic portions outside facing the aqueous environment. Associated with the lipid molecules are globular, amphipathic (i.e., both polar and nonpolar) protein molecules either embedded into or passing through the membrane. The globular proteins may be associated with apparent aqueous pores through which small water-soluble substances may pass.

The proportion of protein and lipid varies with different membranes depending on the membrane function. Some examples are given in Table 3.1. Typically, myelin has insulation properties and a high lipid content, whereas mitochondria are associated with enzyme reactions and have a high protein content.

Table 3.1—Membrane Protein and Lipid Content

Membrane	Protein	Lipid
Myelin	18	79
Human erythrocyte	49	43
Bovine retinal rod	51	49
Mitochondria (outer membrane)	52	48
Mycoplasma laidlawii	58	37
Sarcoplasmic reticulum	67	33
Gram-positive bacteria	75	25
Mitochondria (inner membrane)	76	24

NOTE: All results are percent dry weight.

How do substances cross membranes? In the vast majority of cases, substances cross by passive transfer, which depends on the concentration gradient across the membrane. Fat-soluble compounds tend to cross more readily than water-soluble compounds because membranes are predominantly lipoidal in nature. Weak acids tend to cross membranes more readily when they are in the un-ionized form. The un-ionized form of the acid occurs when the pH of fluids bathing the membrane or at the membrane surface is lower than the pK_a of the acid (5). Weak bases also cross membranes more readily in their un-ionized form. The un-ionized form of the base occurs when the pH of the surrounding fluids is higher than the pK_a of the base.

Both weak acids and weak bases should be absorbed more readily when they are in their un-ionized form. However, to be available for absorption, the drug must also be in solution. A drug cannot pass through a biological membrane in particulate form. Drugs must have some aqueous solubility to dissolve because the GI contents are essentially aqueous. Aqueous solubility is more common for the ionized form of the drug.

Thus, a drug needs to be water-soluble and fat-soluble at the same time for optimal absorption. This problem has plagued pharmaceutical researchers and formulators for a long time.

In practice, it appears that of these two factors, aqueous solubility and membrane crossing, the ability to cross membranes is more important. For example, many fat-soluble drugs are absorbed more readily than their aqueous solubility would predict, and most but not all water-soluble drugs are poorly absorbed. Representative pK_a values of some weakly acidic and weakly basic drugs are given in Table 3.2.

Table 3.2—Ionization Constants (pK_a) of Some Common Acidic and Basic Drugs

Acids		Bases	
Drug	pK_a	*Drug*	pK_a
Cephalothin	2.5	Amphetamine	9.8
Ampicillin	2.5, 7.2	Ephedrine	9.6
Carbenicillin	2.6, 2.7	Imipramine	9.5
Flucloxacillin	2.7	Chlorpromazine	9.3
Methicillin	2.8	Erythromycin	8.8
Probenecid	3.4	Isoprenaline	8.6
Aspirin	3.5	Orphenadrine	8.4
Ibuprofen	4.4	Diphenhydramine	8.3
Chlorpropamide	4.8	Bupivacaine	8.1
Sulfafurazole	4.9	5-Fluorouracil	8.1
Cephalexin	5.2, 7.3	Mepacrine	7.7, 10.3
Dicoumarol	5.7	Codeine	6.0
Nitrofurantoin	7.2	Aminopyrine	5.0
Acetazolamide	7.2	Chlordiazepoxide	4.6
Pentobarbital	8.1	Diazepam	3.3
Phenytoin	8.3	Nitrazepam	3.2, 10.8
Ethosuximide	9.3	Caffeine	0.8

NOTE: Acidic and basic drugs are listed in order of strength. That is, cephalothin is the strongest acid, and ethosuximide is the weakest. Amphetamine is the strongest base, and caffeine is the weakest.

Drugs often cross membranes more efficiently than predicted from simple concentration-gradient concepts and fat-solubility measurements. In these cases, some forms of active or specialized transport have been proposed. Although many types of specialized transport have been described, they can be separated into two major categories, passive facilitated diffusion and active transport. Passive facilitated diffusion is membrane transport driven by a concentration gradient. However, transport is carrier-dependent and saturable. Active transport utilizes cellular energy for drug movement across the membrane, even against a concentration gradient. Transport in this case is saturable and may be reduced by metabolic inhibitors.

Passive facilitated diffusion is a mechanism that is sometimes proposed to explain membrane transport of some water-soluble compounds. For example, the movement of glucose from plasma into red blood cells is a passive process that proceeds with the concentration gradient until equilibrium is reached. At high plasma glucose levels, diffusion across the erythrocyte membrane becomes saturated. Diffusion in this case reaches a form of transport maximum. In common with other carrier-mediated systems, glucose transport is relatively specific and can be inhibited by other molecules. Vitamin B_{12} is also transported across the GI epithelium by passive facilitated diffusion.

Active transport is more common than passive facilitated diffusion but seldom occurs in drug absorption. Examples of active transport are provided by renal and biliary excretion of many acids and bases, and excretion of certain acids from the central nervous system. GI absorption of 5-fluorouracil, riboflavin, and some orally absorbed cephalosporins is thought to occur by active transport. For the great majority of drugs, however, GI absorption appears to occur by passive, concentration-dependent processes.

Physiology of the GI Tract and Its Relationship to Drug Absorption

The GI tract is shown in Figure 3.2. The pH of the region of the mouth, or buccal cavity, is approximately 6.8. Although it is not the most common site for drug absorption, the buccal cavity provides an excellent absorptive environment because it is highly vascular; dense capillary networks are

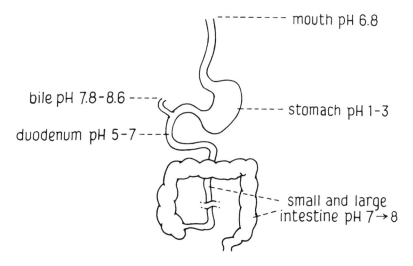

Figure 3.2. The GI tract.

adjacent to the mucous membrane of the buccal cavity and the tongue. The buccal route is used for rapid absorption of drugs, such as nitroglycerin, when rapid effect is required. The buccal cavity is generally only slightly acidic, but the pH of the stomach is about 1–3. This very acidic environment is a consequence of hydrochloric acid secretion by the parietal cells of the stomach. Acid secretion plays an important role in food digestion by facilitating conversion of pepsinogens and zymogens to active proteolytic enzymes. Drug absorption is also profoundly affected.

The acidic environment of the stomach tends to favor absorption of acidic drugs through the gastric epithelium, provided the acidic drugs can dissolve or remain in solution in the acidic fluids of the stomach. On the other hand, basic drugs tend to dissolve quite readily in the stomach, but absorption may be prevented because most of the drug will be in the ionized state and therefore not sufficiently fat-soluble for efficient membrane transport to occur.

The acidic environment of the stomach may also cause reduced drug bioavailability because of acid-catalyzed degradation. Many organic bases are unstable in acid and undergo rapid chemical degradation unless they are protected in some way. An example of this kind of organic base is the antibiotic erythromycin. Erythromycin is used for a variety of infections commonly associated with Gram-positive organisms. Erythromycin is efficiently absorbed from oral doses and is generally administered by that route, although an intravenous form does exist. Erythromycin is a base and is susceptible to acid-catalyzed degradation in the stomach that may lead to poor and erratic absorption.

Two approaches have been taken to prevent erythromycin degradation. The first approach is to formulate erythromycin base or its stearate salt in tablets or capsules that have acid-resistant coatings. With this type of formulation, the coating remains intact while the tablet or capsule is in the acidic environment of the stomach, but the coating dissolves to release active ingredient after the tablet passes from the stomach into the relatively alkaline small intestine.

The second approach to prevent degradation is to convert erythromycin to an acid-stable esterified derivative. The esterified forms of erythromycin are also more lipophilic than the parent drug and can cross the membranes of the GI epithelium more efficiently. Examples of erythromycin esters currently in clinical use are erythromycin ethylsuccinate and erythromycin estolate, the latter being the lauryl sulfate salt of the propionyl ester of erythromycin. These esters of erythromycin are so stable and insoluble in water that they can be formulated as suspension dosage forms that are particularly useful in pediatric therapy.

If a drug dissolves in the stomach or is a liquid, and if it is fat-soluble and acid-stable, then the drug is likely to be absorbed efficiently from the stomach. A good example of this kind of drug is ethyl alcohol. Alcohol is normally a liquid that is completely miscible with water, sufficiently lipophilic to cross membranes, and therefore efficiently absorbed from the stomach.

Because the absorptive properties of the proximal small intestine are so superior to those of the stomach, or any other part of the GI tract, alcohol and most other compounds are more efficiently absorbed from the proximal small intestine region. To reach the small intestine, drug must pass through the pyloric sphincter, which separates the stomach from the duodenum, and the rate at which this occurs is a function of stomach emptying. Thus, the rate at which substances pass from the stomach into the small intestine is one of the major rate-limiting steps controlling drug absorption.

Stomach motility is a complex phenomenon that is influenced by a variety of nervous and hormonal stimuli. Stomach-emptying rate is a function of rhythmic contractions. These contractions, which are quite vigorous, have a frequency of approximately three per minute in a hungry person and become diminished when food enters the stomach. Food passes from the stomach through the pyloric sphincter into the duodenum as a result of these rhythmic contractions. The heavier the meal and the higher the fat content, the longer it will take for the meal and any drug ingested with the meal to pass into the small intestine. The reduced number of contractions and force of gastric rhythms, and the consequent decrease in gastric emptying rate after meals, appear to result from nervous and hormonal feedback mechanisms that are due to activation of receptors situated in the duodenum, the fat receptors, osmoreceptors, and acid receptors. This finely tuned process can be regarded as a defense mechanism in which substances are prevented from entering the proximal small intestine and injuring the delicate absorptive surface of that region until the substances have been reduced to a suitable consistency in the stomach.

Although solid food tends to delay stomach emptying, liquids tend to speed the process. In fact, increased fluid volume is the only known natural stimulus to stomach emptying. This stimulation results from activation of stretch receptors in the stomach wall. When the fluid is water, subsequent activation of the inhibitory receptors in the duodenum is stopped, and the net result is rapid emptying of the stomach contents. From a physical viewpoint, drugs should be absorbed better from concentrated solutions than from diluted solutions because of a greater concentration gradient. However, the reverse is often the case. Studies in experimental animals and humans have shown that drug absorption from the GI tract increases when drug is administered as a solid dosage form or as a solution, when the drug is in a large fluid volume. This increased drug absorption results from the combined effects of accelerated stomach emptying, rapid exposure of dissolved drug molecules to a larger GI surface area, and faster dissolution of solid dosage forms.

After passing through the pyloric sphincter, drug reaches the duodenum and then the jejunum and the ileum. These regions of the GI tract differ from the stomach with respect to pH, the presence of digestive enzymes, and the absorptive surface area.

Excretion of alkaline bile, which has a pH of 7.8–8.6, into the duodenum raises the pH of the duodenal and subsequent intestinal contents to approximately 5–7. Bile salts, which are surface-active, promote dissolution of lipophilic drugs and also lipophilic drug formulations, enteric coatings, and waxy drug matrices. Bile salts may also promote membrane permeability of hydrophobic molecules through micelle formation and solubilization. On the other hand, bile salts have been known to form insoluble complexes with some drugs including neomycin, kanamycin, and vancomycin. Insoluble complex formation could reduce systemic availability of these drugs.

Proteolytic enzymes are secreted into the duodenum. Protein or polypeptide drugs such as corticotropin, vasopressin, and insulin are rapidly degraded by intestinal enzymes and cannot be given orally. The hormonal agents progesterone, testosterone, and aldosterone are similarly unstable in the intestine and are generally given by the buccal route or by parenteral routes.

The abrupt change of pH from acidic to neutral on passing from the stomach into the proximal small intestine causes many changes. Enteric coatings that were impermeable in the stomach will dissolve. Acidic drugs will also dissolve in the relatively basic environment, and the pH will not be raised sufficiently to prevent dissolution or cause precipitation of most weakly basic drugs.

By far the most important difference between the proximal small intestine and the stomach is the nature of the mucosal surface of the epithelium. As shown in Figure 3.3, the mucosal surface of the small intestine has a unique morphology because its surface area is increased by finger-like projections, or villi, arising from the folds of Kerckring, which are folds in the intestinal mucosa, and by microvilli in turn arising from the villi. These various invaginations and projections increase the surface area of the mucosa approximately 600-fold. The total surface area of the small intestine has been calculated to be approximately 200 m^2, and an estimated 1–1.5 L of blood pass through the intestinal capillaries each minute. The corresponding values for the stomach are only 100 m^2 of surface area, and a blood flow rate of 150 mL/min. Thus, the intestine has a surface area approximately double that of the stomach but a blood perfusion rate that is 6–10 times faster. Both factors—surface area and blood perfusion rate—strongly favor more efficient absorption from the intestine than from the stomach.

The villi and microvilli of the intestine, like many other cells in the body, are lined by a sulfated mucoprotein, glycocalyx, also known as the fuzzy-coat. Fluid that is trapped within the glycocalyx is stationary, and a series of thin layers, each progressively more stirred, extends from the

STRUCTURE	INCREASE IN SURFACE AREA (relative to cylinder)	SURFACE AREA (sq. cm.)
AREA OF SIMPLE CYLINDER	1	3,300
FOLDS OF KERKRING	3	10,000
VILLI	30	100,000
MICROVILLI	600	2,000,000

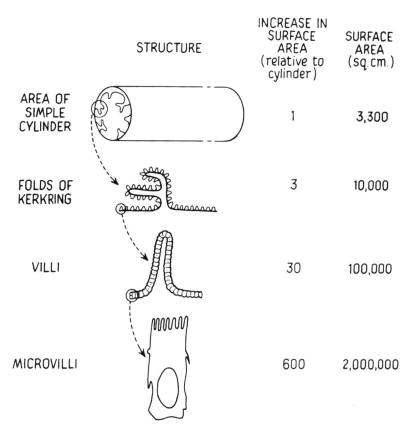

Figure 3.3. Anatomical features that influence the surface area of the small intestine. (Reproduced with permission from reference 3. Copyright 1962, W. B. Saunders.)

epithelial cell surface to the bulk phase of the intestinal lumen. This series of thin layers is known as the "unstirred layer" and has an effective thickness of 0.01–1.0 mm.

Molecules move within the unstirred layer only by diffusion because there is no convection. The rate of diffusion is inversely proportional to the square root of molecular weight below 450, and inversely proportional to the cube root of molecular weight above 450.

The glycocalyx on the microvilli is negatively charged and the counterions are in the unstirred layer. If a substantial portion of these cations is composed of hydrogen ions, as is often the case, then the microclimate within the brush border of the epithelium is likely to be acidic relative to the bulk phase of the intestinal lumen. This may influence drug ionization at the membrane surface and may provide a basis for the "acid microclimate" frequently associated with the GI mucosa.

The length of time during which material stays in the small intestine varies, but a reasonable estimate is 5 min in the duodenum, 2 h in the jejeunum, and 3–6 h in the ileum. After passing through these regions, material then enters the large intestine.

The large intestine is similar to the stomach because it does not have villi or microvilli at its mucosal surface, but it is different from the stomach in terms of pH. The stomach contents are strongly acidic, but the large intestine tends to be neutral or alkaline. Absorption of drugs from the large intestine tends to be less efficient compared with the small intestine. The large intestine and colon contain an active bacterial microflora. This microflora is capable of degrading foreign molecules and will tend to reduce the availability of drugs present in this region of the GI tract.

At the extreme distal end of the GI tract is the rectum. The rectum contains no microvilli and apparently no sites for active absorption, has an active bacterial microflora, and usually contains fecal material. Combination of these factors would suggest that the rectum is a very poor absorption site. However, absorption is not necessarily poor. Drugs are frequently administered in the form of suppositories or enemas, and absorption efficiency is often good, if erratic. Some drugs given rectally for systemic action include acetaminophin, aspirin, indomethacin, perchlorperazine, phenobarbital, promethazine, and theophylline.

Once a drug crosses from the mucosal to the serosal side of the GI epithelium, the drug may be transported away from the serosal side by one or both of two mechanisms. The GI tract is bathed by a blood–capillary network that is associated with the splanchnic circulation. This network is close to the GI epithelium and provides a perfect route for drug absorption. In addition to the blood supply, the GI tract is also extensively supplied by the lymphatic system. Therefore, absorbed material could also be taken up by the lymphatic vessels in the GI epithelium and carried in the lymphatic system that drains the abdominal area to the thoracic duct. The absorbed material could then join the venous system of the general circulation at the junction of the left internal jugular vein and the subclavian vein. Despite the presence of the blood–capillary network and lymphatic system, absorption of the great majority of drugs appears to occur almost exclusively via the capillary system associated with the splanchnic circulation.

Why should GI drug absorption be so selective for the splanchnic circulation? The answer appears to lie in the relative flow rate of blood and lymph. The rate of blood flow in the splanchnic circulation bathing the abdominal area is 1–1.5 L min^{-1}, and this rate represents approximately 30% of cardiac output. This rate may increase to 2 L/min after a meal. Lymph flow through the same region is only 1–2 mL/min, although this may increase to 5–20 mL/min after a meal. Lymph flow in this region thus is approximately 500–700 times slower than blood flow. The relatively fast splanchnic bloodflow establishes virtually sink conditions on the serosal side of the GI epithelium and a very steep concentration gradient across the membrane. These conditions promote efficient absorption into the bloodstream. This situation does not exist with very sluggish lymph flow. Therefore, from purely physical viewpoints, efficient absorption associated with splanchnic circulation would not be expected via the lymphatic system.

For most drugs, absorption from the GI tract occurs via the bloodstream. Only a very small fraction of drug molecules may be absorbed via the lymphatic system. These include drugs with very high molecular weights that have difficulty entering the capillaries, and also some specific molecules such as steroids.

The routes of drug absorption from all regions of the GI tract into the bloodstream are shown in Figure 3.4. The left side of the figure represents the regions of the GI tract, and the right side represents the systemic circulation. The continuous arrows running horizontally from the GI tract to the systemic circulation indicate that substances absorbed from these regions enter the systemic circulation directly via the capillary networks. Drug absorption from the buccal cavity, for example, occurs into the dense vascular network in the oral mucosa that leads into the superior vena cava. Absorption from the lower rectum occurs via the inferior and middle hemorrhoidal veins that lead directly into the inferior vena cava.

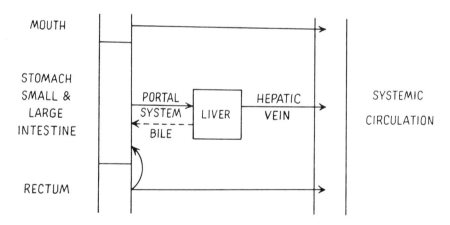

Figure 3.4. Routes by which substances may pass from the GI tract into the systemic circulation.

Only from the buccal cavity and lower rectum are compounds absorbed directly into the systemic circulation. Compounds absorbed from any other region of the GI tract, stomach, small intestine, large intestine, colon, and upper rectum enter the capillary networks associated with the splanchnic circulation. The splanchnic circulation leads into the portal vein. The portal vein leads into the liver and subsequently to the hepatic vein that leads into the general circulation at the junction with the inferior vena cava. Thus, the vast majority of drugs must pass through the liver during absorption. This first pass through the liver is an extremely important process that may limit the absorption of certain drugs. This process is important for the following reasons:

1. During the brief time period during which drug is being transported from the GI tract via the capillaries of the splanchnic circulation until it mixes with the general circulation at the inferior vena cava, drug is confined to the volume of the splanchnic circulation and has not yet distributed into the rest of the vascular system, nor to other body tissues and fluids into which it may eventually partition. Therefore, during the first pass through the liver, drug is at a higher concentration than it will be after it has mixed with other parts of the vascular system and other body tissues and fluids.

2. The liver is the principal organ for drug metabolism.

3. Drug metabolism is generally a first-order process. Thus, the higher the concentration of drug presented to the liver, the greater the quantity of drug metabolized.

Consider the combined effect of points 1–3. Drug molecules that are absorbed from the GI tract are confined to the splanchnic circulation and are presented to the metabolizing enzymes of the liver at a high concentration during the first pass. This step is illustrated in Figure 3.5. If hepatic metabolism is assumed to be first-order in nature, then a certain proportion of drug will be removed by the liver during the first pass, depending on the hepatic extraction ratio, and reduced drug availability to

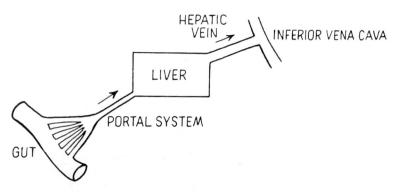

Figure 3.5. Absorption via the splanchnic circulation.

the general circulation results. The greater the extent and efficiency of hepatic extraction, the larger the proportion of absorbed drug removed by the liver and the greater the first-pass effect.

The first-pass effect is likely to be important for any orally administered drug that is extensively metabolized and has a high hepatic extraction ratio. A drug may be very efficiently absorbed from the GI tract and yet may be poorly absorbed into the general circulation because of this second line of defense. Little or no first-pass effect will occur if a drug undergoes little or no hepatic metabolism.

Summary

1. Stomach-emptying rate may influence drug absorption and GI residence time in general.

2. Other factors that may influence drug absorption include secretion of acid, bile, and digestive enzymes; the unstirred layer; the glycocalyx; and drug degradation by intestinal microflora.

3. Drugs may be absorbed from the GI tract via the splanchnic circulation or via the lymphatic system. The splanchnic route is the most efficient but is accompanied by the potential problem of first-pass hepatic metabolism.

Literature Cited

1. Davenport, H. W. *Physiology of the Digestive Tract*, 4th ed.; Year Book Medical Publishers: Chicago, 1978.
2. Bates, T. R.; Gibaldi, M. In *Current Concepts in the Pharmaceutical Sciences: Biopharmaceutics*; Swarbrick, J., Ed.; Lea and Febiger: Philadelphia, 1970; 57–99.
3. Wilson, T. H. *Intestinal Absorption*; Saunders: Philadelphia, 1962, 2.
4. Singer, S. J.; Nicolson, G. L. *Science* **1972,** *175,* 720–731.
5. Hogben, C. A. M.; Tocco, D. J.; Brodie, B. B.; Schanker, L. S. *J. Pharmacol. Exp. Ther.* **1959,** *125,* 275–282.

4

First-Pass Metabolism, Enterohepatic Circulation, and Physicochemical Factors Affecting Absorption

First-Pass Metabolism

The problem of first-pass metabolism was identified in Chapter 3. It was established that for drugs that are efficiently cleared by the liver, first-pass metabolism can result in poor drug availability to the systemic circulation despite the fact that the drug may be efficiently absorbed from the GI lumen into the splanchnic circulation.

Several methods have been described that predict the degree of first-pass metabolism of an orally administered compound. Two of the original methods were by Gibaldi et al. (*1*) and Rowland (*2*). One of several possible approaches based on the hepatic extraction ratio will be described here. The oral availability of a drug that undergoes extensive hepatic metabolism can be predicted with this approach from Equation 4.1

$$\text{oral availability} = 1 - E_H \qquad (4.1)$$

where E_H is the hepatic extraction ratio. Clearly if E_H is 0, then the liver does not extract, no metabolism occurs, and all of the drug that is ab-

0065–7719/86/0185–0035$06.00/1
© 1986 American Chemical Society

sorbed from the GI tract may reach the systemic circulation. On the other hand, if E_H is 1, that is, all of the drug is extracted during each pass through the liver, then the oral availability is likely to be 0. Complete hepatic extraction of drug may occur despite very efficient absorption from the GI tract into the splanchnic circulation.

Equation 4.1 introduces the problem of determining the magnitude of the extraction ratio. This value has been described for many drugs, but one method by which it can be measured is by means of Equation 4.2.

$$E_H = \frac{\text{hepatic clearance}}{\text{hepatic blood flow}} \tag{4.2}$$

where hepatic clearance is the volume of blood that is cleared of drug by the liver per unit time, in milliliters per minute; and blood flow is equivalent to splanchnic blood supply to the liver via the portal vein, which is approximately 1200 mL/min. The hepatic clearance can also be calculated after intravenous doses from Equation 4.3, where the dose is the intravenous dose, and $AUC^{0 \to \infty}$ is the area under the blood-concentration curve from zero to infinite time.

$$\text{hepatic clearance} = \frac{\text{dose}}{AUC^{0 \to \infty}} \tag{4.3}$$

A mathematical example will help to illustrate this method of predicting the hepatic extraction ratio. Suppose that a 100-mg dose of an extensively metabolized drug was administered by intravenous injection, and the area under the blood-concentration versus time curve is 280 μg/min/mL. To maintain consistency in units, the dose is multiplied by 1000 to express it in micrograms. Dividing the dose by the area under the curve as in Equation 4.3 yields 357 mL/min. This value is the hepatic clearance. Hepatic clearance can then be divided by hepatic blood flow as in Equation 4.2. The clearance is 357 mL/min, and if hepatic blood flow is, for example, 1200 mL/min, then the hepatic extraction ratio is 0.298, or 0.3. From Equation 4.1, the oral bioavailability is 0.7, or 70%. This value represents the best availability one might expect because the calculations assume that all of the drug is absorbed from the GI tract into the splanchnic circulation.

This type of approach is useful to predict the systemic availability of oral drug doses, but it also provides additional information. Consider the example again and recall that it predicts that drug availability to the general circulation should not exceed 70%, provided that the drug is efficiently absorbed from the GI tract into the splanchnic circulation. This hypothesis can be tested by giving the drug orally and actually measuring the systemic availability by comparing areas under blood-concentration curves from oral and intravenous doses. If the actual bioavailability is approximately 70%, then the prediction method is accurate (or at least appears to be). If the bioavailability value is less than 70%, then the drug probably was not efficiently absorbed from the GI tract because of a stability problem, poor solubility, an inappropriate formulation, or because the drug may not cross the GI epithelium very efficiently. For example, if the observed availability was actually 35%, then one can conclude that only 50% of the drug was absorbed into the splanchnic circulation.

The other possible situation is for the observed value to be greater than the predicted value. Although 70% bioavailability is predicted from the previous example, the actual availability may be 80% or 90% based on the relative area values from oral and intravenous doses. This situation is somewhat more difficult to interpret than the previous one. Certainly, the low predicted value is not related to GI absorption because the calculations assumed this value to be 100%. The only possible explanation relates to the degree of first-pass metabolism. The prediction method assumes first-order metabolism. However, if metabolism is not first-order but is saturable at high drug concentrations, which is more likely to occur during the first pass than at other times, then the actual hepatic extraction ratio E_H will decrease and systemic availability will be greater than predicted. Drugs that have intermediate hepatic extraction ratios include aspirin, codeine, nortriptyline, and quinidine (3). Drugs that have high extraction ratios include

- alprenolol
- arabinosylcytosine
- desipramine
- fluorouracil
- isoproterenol
- lidocaine
- meperidine
- morphine
- pentazocine
- propoxyphene
- propranolol
- salicylamide

Enterohepatic Circulation

The human liver secretes between 500 mL and 1 L of bile each day into the duodenum via the gall bladder and the common bile duct. Bile contains bile salts that have a solubilizing effect and thus promote the absorption of fats.

Approximately 90% of bile salts and bile acids that are secreted in bile are reabsorbed from the intestine and return to the liver where they are again available for secretion. A schematic diagram of this system is given in Figure 4.1. By means of this continuous secretion process, these

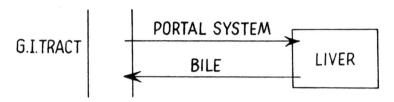

Figure 4.1. Enterohepatic circulation. A schematic of biliary excretion and reabsorption.

compounds undergo enterohepatic circulation, which is a term that describes continuous recirculation between the liver and the intestine. This closed loop system is very efficient because it enables bile salts and acids to be used many times. Enterohepatic cycling can also occur with drugs and other foreign compounds.

Biliary excretion is similar to renal tubular secretion (Chapter 9) because biliary excretion occurs by an active, energy-consuming process and can transport substances against a considerable concentration gradient. The ability of a drug to be excreted in bile is related to its chemical structure and molecular weight (4). Different species exhibit different molecular weight thresholds, which is the minimum molecular weight necessary to be excreted in the bile. For example, the rat has a lower molecular weight threshold of approximately 200 for biliary excretion of quaternary ammonium compounds and about 300 for aromatic anions. Humans, on the other hand, have a lower molecular weight threshold of 300 for quaternary ammonium compounds and over 400 for most other compounds.

Drugs can be excreted in bile in unchanged form or as metabolized conjugates. The metabolized conjugate form is favored if conjugation brings the molecular weight of the compound above the minimum threshold value. To be excreted in unchanged form, drugs must meet the molecular weight criterion and also contain a polar functional group such as ammonium, carboxyl, or sulfate.

If after being excreted in the bile into the duodenum the compound or its metabolites are not reabsorbed, then they are voided in the feces or further degraded by bacterial microflora, and the bile becomes an efficient elimination route. However, the unchanged drug or deconjugated metabolites, which exist because of the action of intestinal enzymes or intestinal bacterial degradation, can be reabsorbed into the bloodstream and thus set up a similar type of enterohepatic cycle to that of the bile salts. Compounds such as cromolyn sodium, erythromycin, and rifampin are excreted unchanged in bile. Conversely, compounds such as carbenoxolone, estradiol, indomethacin, and morphine are excreted in the bile mainly as conjugates. The new cephalosporin, cefoperazone, undergoes extensive biliary excretion in humans. This route of excretion accounts for 60–70% of total eliminated drug, and concentrations of cefoperazone in bile may be 10 to 20 times higher than those in serum (5,6). The degree to which enterohepatic cycling occurs with many compounds in humans is not known with any certainty. This uncertainty arises mainly because most human biliary excretion data have to be obtained during gall bladder surgery, and information is scanty for most compounds.

As noted previously, drugs can be extensively metabolized in the liver during the first pass. Because bile formation also initiates in the liver, and because drugs are taken up by bile in that organ, drugs that are extensively excreted in bile will also have their systemic absorption reduced by this process in addition to any hepatic metabolism. Therefore, any drug extensively metabolized and excreted in bile is in double jeopardy and is unlikely to exhibit good systemic availability regardless of possibly good GI absorption.

The exact nature of the enterohepatic cycle may be complex because hepatic extraction occurs from blood supplied by both the portal and hepatic veins. Thus, the recycling process involves drug that is just entering the body via the splanchnic circulation and also drug that is passing through the liver from both the portal and hepatic veins as part of the general systemic circulation. Whatever processes are involved, biliary recycling, or the enterohepatic cycle, can prolong the apparent elimination rate of a drug.

Prolonged drug existence has been elegantly demonstrated for the cardiac drug digitoxin. Oral maintenance doses of cholestyramine were administered orally 8 h after a dose of tritiated digitoxin. Cholestyramine is a nonabsorbable ion-exchange resin capable of binding digitoxin and some of its metabolites in the intestine and thereby preventing their absorption or reabsorption. Cholestyramine treatment caused a marked reduction in the elimination half-life of radioactivity in serum from 11.5 to 6.6 days, and this reduction was presumably the result of cholestyramine preventing reabsorption of biliary excreted digitoxin or its metabolites.

Physicochemical Factors Affecting Absorption

The chemical and physical properties of a drug are of primary concern to the formulator because these characteristics can affect drug stability, absorption characteristics, and ease of formulation.

A variety of chemical options can be used to improve the stability and absorption of a drug without affecting its pharmacological properties. For example, erythromycin can be esterified to produce more acid-stable and fat-soluble derivatives for improved oral availability. The esters do not appear to be bacteriologically active, but they become active when they are hydrolyzed back to the free base. Another example of this type of drug is hetacillin, which is hydrolyzed to the active form ampicillin during or after absorption.

Both the stability and solubility of weak acids and bases are increased or tend to be increased when in the form of water-soluble salts. Figure 4.2 shows how administration of soluble salts of pencillin V results in

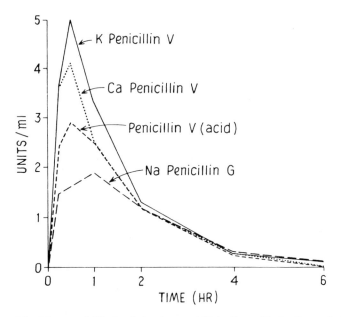

Figure 4.2. Mean penicillin levels in plasma of 10 fasting subjects after oral administration of four doses of 105 units of penicillin in different forms. (Reproduced with permission from reference 8. Copyright 1971, Hoffmann-LaRoche, Inc.)

higher plasma levels compared to the free acid (7). The high levels of the potassium salt compared to the calcium salt are consistent with their relative aqueous solubilities and therefore their dissolution rate in the GI tract. The low levels obtained from penicillin G sodium are due to this penicillin being less stable in gastric juice compared to penicillin V. The rationale for better absorption of the water-soluble salts of penicillin compared to the free acid form is described in Figure 4.3. The pH of a solution of a strong base and a weak acid, which is what the penicillin salts and the salts of most acidic drugs are, is given by Equation 4.4.

$$pH = 0.5(pK_w + pK_a + \log C) \tag{4.4}$$

where pK_w is the negative logarithm of the dissociation constant for water, pK_a is the negative logarithm of the dissociation constant for the weak

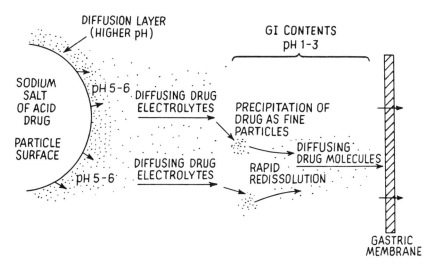

Figure 4.3. Schematic diagram of dissolution process in the stomach from the surface of a water-soluble salt of a relatively insoluble weak acid. (Reproduced with permission from reference 8. Copyright 1971, Hoffmann-LaRoche, Inc.)

acid, and C is the molar concentration of total weak acid. For a weak acid with a pK_a of 2.8, which is the approximate pK_a for most penicillins, and a concentration of 1 M, Equation 4.4 becomes Equation 4.5.

$$pH = 0.5(14 + 2.8 + 0) = 8.4 \qquad (4.5)$$

Equation 4.5 shows that the drug solution will have an alkaline reaction. Applying this concept to Figure 4.3 shows that as the sodium salt of the acidic drug dissolves in the stomach, the salt generates a diffusion layer of relatively high pH that will in turn promote further dissolution of the weak acid. As the dissolved molecules move into the bulk stomach contents, the pH will fall and may cause drug precipitation. If drug precipitation does occur, the drug will precipitate in very fine particles that will tend to redissolve readily (8).

The same argument could be used for basic drugs, but the pH effect resulting from the use of salts of weak bases is far less important because this effect will be swamped by the low pH of the stomach. Thus, salts of basic drugs are used primarily to ease handling and stability and are less important for improved dissolution.

Physical Factors Affecting Absorption

Different physical forms of a drug can be used to improve or optimize absorption. Typically, the crystal or polymorphic form of a drug, the state or form of hydration or solvation, and the physical size of drug particles can be varied often with considerable effect on drug absorption characteristics.

Polymorphism and Amorphism. Many compounds can form crystals with different molecular arrangements, or *polymorphs*. While these polymorphs have identical chemistry, they may have different physical properties such as melting point, dissolution rate, and overall solubility. For example, the vitamin riboflavin exists in a number of polymorphic forms, and these forms have a 20-fold range in aqueous solubility. Polymorphs that have no crystal structure, or amorphic forms, have different physical characteristics than the crystalline form.

Different polymorphs of organic compounds, including the amorphic form, may be produced depending on temperature, solvent of crystallization, and other factors during their preparation. Often one polymorph will be the most stable, and other forms will tend to convert to that form at a rate and an extent depending on prevailing conditions.

The most important effect that polymorphism has in pharmacokinetics is on dissolution. Absorption of many orally administered drugs is dissolution rate controlled. According to the Noyes–Whitney solution rate law, amorphous forms of a drug dissolve faster than crystalline forms because no energy is required to break up the crystal lattice. Thus, from the standpoint of the rate and (often) the extent of absorption, the amorphous form is preferred over crystalline forms and several drugs, including chloramphenicol palmitate, hydrocortisone, and prednisolone are marketed in their amorphous forms. An interesting example of the use of combined polymorphs to provide optimal therapeutic effect is provided by insulin, where a mixture of amorphous and crystalline forms provides initial fast release from the amorphous component and sustained release from the crystalline component.

Solvation. During their preparation, drug crystals may incorporate one or more solvent molecules to form solvates. The type of solvate formed can influence drug dissolution rate. The most common solvate is water. If water molecules are already present in a crystal structure, then the tendency for the crystal to attract additional water to initiate the dissolution process is reduced, and solvated (in this case hydrated) crystalline forms tend to dissolve more slowly than anhydrous forms. Although solvation was originally considered to be important for some drugs such as ampicillin, observed differences in drug absorption from hydrated and anhydrous drug forms are not great and are generally clinically significant. Significant differences have been observed in the dissolution of hydrated and anhydrous forms of caffeine, theophylline, glutethimide, and mercaptopurine. The significance of these differences regarding in vivo absorption has not been examined but is likely to be slight as with ampicillin.

Particle Size. Unlike solvation, particle size can play a major role in the absorption of slowly dissolving drugs (9). The dissolution rate of solid particles is proportional to surface area, and surface area is related to the fineness of the particle. Particle size reduction has been used to increase the absorption of a large number of poorly soluble drugs such as

- bishydroxycoumarin
- chloramphenicol
- digoxin
- griseofulvin
- medroxyprogesterone acetate

- nitrofurantoin
- phenobarbital
- phenacetin
- spironolactone
- tolbutamide

Griseofulvin is an interesting member of this group. This drug is a potent fungicide that is taken orally. Griseofulvin has extremely low aqueous solubility, and material of normal particle size results in poor and erratic absorption. Absorption was greatly improved when microsize particles were prepared, but was improved even more when the drug was formulated in ultramicrosize particles as a monomolecular dispersion (solid solution) in poly(ethylene glycol) 6000.

Summary

1. First-pass metabolism may be important for extensively metabolized drugs, or drugs that are extensively cleared in the bile. First-pass metabolism occurs from all GI absorption sites except the mouth and the lower rectum. It may also occur after intraperitoneal dosage because much of the drug administered by this route is absorbed via the splanchnic circulation. A method was described to predict the first-pass effect from intravenous data, and the implications of deviations from predicted values with this method were considered.

2. Biliary excretion and the enterohepatic cycle can influence the absorption of drugs and the elimination of drugs that are subjected to these phenomena.

3. Chemical and physical factors may influence drug absorption characteristics. Most of the factors including ester and salt formation, polymorphism, solvation, and particle size affect drug stability and dissolution. Particle size is frequently rate-limiting for in vivo absorption of many drugs.

Literature Cited

1. Gibaldi, M.; Boyes, R. N.; Feldman, S. *J. Pharm. Sci.* **1971,** *60,* 1338–1340.
2. Rowland, M. *J. Pharm. Sci.* **1972,** *61,* 71–74.
3. Rowland, M.; Tozer, T. *Clinical Pharmacokinetics: Concepts and Applications;* Lea & Febiger: Philadelphia, 1980; 51.
4. Smith, R. L. *Handb. Exp. Pharmacol.* **1971,** *28,* 354–389.
5. Craig, W. A.; Gerber, A. U.; Barbhaiya, R. H.; Welling, P. G. *Abstracts of Papers,* Cefoperazone Symposium, New Orleans, 1980, Excerpta Medica.
6. Shimizy, K. *Clin. Ther.,* **1980,** *3,* 60–79.
7. Juncher, H.; Raaschou, F. *Antibiot. Med. Clin. Ther.* **1957,** *4,* 497–507.
8. Cadwallader, D. E. *Biopharmaceutics and Drug Interactions;* Roche Scientific Monographs; Hoffmann-LaRoche: Nutley, NJ, 1971; 65.
9. Niazi, S. *Textbook of Biopharmaceutics and Clinical Pharmacokinetics;* Appleton–Century–Crofts: New York, 1979; 28–30.

Problems

1. Following a 100-mg intravenous bolus dose of a drug that equilibrates evenly between plasma and blood red cells, the area under the plasma curve ($AUC^{0 \to \infty}$) is calculated to be 250 μg/min/mL. Assuming that the hepatic blood flow rate is 1200 mL/min, predict the maximum systemic availability of the drug after an oral dose.

2. If the actual observed systemic availability of the oral dose was only 33%, what is the absorption efficiency of the drug from the GI tract into the splanchnic circulation?

5

Formulation Factors Affecting Drug Absorption

Drug formulations are designed to provide a product that is attractive, distinctive, convenient to use, stable, and has the appropriate physico-chemical characteristics to provide an optimal absorption profile. Although the importance of the first four factors is acknowledged, only the appropriate physicochemical characteristics for optimum absorption are considered here. Currently available conventional dosage forms, in order of increasing dissolution rate, are controlled-release formulations, coated tablets, tablets, capsules, suspensions, solid solutions, and solutions (1).

Solutions

Aqueous solutions in the form of elixirs, syrups, emulsions, or just simple solutions do not have a dissolution problem and generally result in faster and more complete absorption of passively absorbed drugs (i.e., the overwhelming majority of drugs) compared to other dosage forms. Some acidic drugs administered as water-soluble salts may precipitate in the acidic pH of stomach fluids, but such precipitates, as described in the previous chapter, are likely to be in finely divided form and should readily redissolve either within the stomach or as they pass into the relatively alkaline environment of the small intestine. Because of the ease with which these acidic drugs can be swallowed, solution dosage forms are particularly useful for pediatric or geriatric patients and for patients who may have difficulty swallowing solid dosage forms. Solutions are the best

0065–7719/86/0185–0045$06.00/1
© 1986 American Chemical Society

dosage forms for oral bioavailability and are frequently used as standards against which other oral dosage forms are compared.

Although most oral solutions are aqueous, nonaqueous solutions or emulsions may be useful in particular cases. For example, a solution of indoxole in oil, as an oil-in-water emulsion, is absorbed three times more efficiently than an aqueous solution.

Solid Solutions

The solid solution is a novel formulation approach in which drug is trapped as a solid solution or molecular dispersion in a water-soluble matrix that leads to a very large surface area to interact with GI fluids. Although the solid solution method is an attractive approach, particularly for lipophilic molecules that have dissolution and bioavailability problems, only one drug, griseofulvin, is currently marketed in this form (*see* Chapter 4).

Suspensions

A drug that is formulated as a suspension is in solid form, but the drug is finely divided, has a large surface area, and is freely available to interact with, and dissolve in, the GI fluids. The drug particles can also disperse and diffuse readily between the stomach and small intestine so that absorption of suspensions is likely to be less sensitive to stomach-emptying rate than other solid dosage forms.

Besides the esters of erythromycin that were already discussed in relation to chemical drug manipulation in Chapter 3, many other antimicrobial agents are administered in suspension forms. These suspension-form drugs include chloramphenicol palmitate, some penicillins, tetracyclines, nitrofurantoin, and sulfonamides.

Similar to solutions, suspensions are useful dosage forms for patients who experience difficulty with solid medication. Adjusting the dose to a patient's exact requirements is easier with solutions and suspensions than with solid dosage forms. (An exception is solid solutions that are marketed as compressed tablets.) Giving one-half or two-thirds of a tablet or a fraction of a capsule may be difficult. Liquid dosage forms therefore have practical advantages besides simple dissolution effects. However, liquid dosage forms also have disadvantages; the principal ones are greater bulk, difficulty of handling, and often reduced stability compared to solid products.

Capsules and Tablets

Capsules and tablets are the most commonly used oral dosage forms. These two types of formulations differ in that material in capsules is less impacted than in compressed tablets. Once the capsule dissolves, the encapsulated material can disperse quickly in a manner similar to a suspension. The capsule material, although water-soluble, can impede drug dissolution by interacting with drug material, but this interaction is uncommon.

The processes leading to tablet disintegration, dissolution, and absorption are described in Figure 5.1 (2). Tablets generally disintegrate in stages, first into granules and then into primary particles. As particle size decreases, dissolution rate increases because of increased surface area.

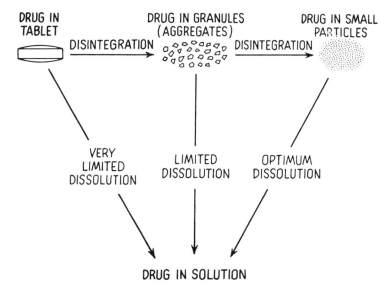

Figure 5.1. Tablet disintegration and dissolution. (Reproduced with permission from reference 2. Copyright 1971, Hoffmann-LaRoche, Inc.)

At one time, tablet disintegration into granules or into primary particles was considered to be a sufficient criterion to predict in vivo absorption. However, now dissolution is recognized as a better criterion and bears a closer, albeit tenuous, relationship with in vivo absorption rates.

Regulatory agencies now require dissolution data for new formulations. The increasingly wide acceptance of dissolution as the best available in vitro parameter to establish drug uniformity and drug release rate, and to predict in vivo absorption, is reflected in the proliferation of such tests in official compendia. For example, the 1975 *United States Pharmacopeia and National Formulary* combined contained dissolution tests for some 20 drug products. The 1980 *Pharmacopeia*, on the other hand, contained 53 such tests, and tests for an additional 217 products have appeared in subsequent supplements to the *Pharmacopeia*.

Along with active substance or substances contained in tablets and capsules, a variety of so-called inert ingredients are present. For example, tablets and capsules may contain magnesium stearate or talc to improve flow properties. Starch, magnesium aluminum silicate, methylcellulose, carboxymethylcellulose, or acacia may be present as binders or disintegrants. Lactose, kaolin, calcium sulfate, magnesium stearate, or other materials may be found as simple bulk agents and diluents. Tablets may also incorporate a variety of coatings to improve their stability, taste, appearance, and release characteristics. Although considered to be inert, these additives can affect drug dissolution and absorption. For example, changing the excipient (or diluent) from calcium sulfate to lactose and increasing the content of magnesium silicate increased the activity of oral phenytoin. The systemic availability of thiamine and riboflavin was reduced by the presence of Fuller's earth, which adsorbs these drugs. Similarly, absorption of tetracycline from capsules is reduced by calcium phosphate because of complex formation.

Most of these interactions were reported some time ago, and the present level of sophistication associated with the pharmaceutical industry suggests that these interactions are unlikely to occur today. However, as recently as 1971, different formulations of digoxin yielded up to sevenfold differences in serum levels (3). This example may be taken as an object lesson never to underestimate the potential of excipient-drug interactions to increase or decrease drug absorption.

Coated Tablets

Tablets are often formulated with a coating, usually some form of acid-insoluble material such as shellac, resin, or styrene–maleic acid copolymer. Coated tablets are insoluble at acidic pH but dissolve readily at neutral or alkaline pH. Coated tablets are therefore ideally suited to prevent release of drug in the stomach, and yet permit release of drug after the dosage form has left the stomach and entered the relatively alkaline region of the small intestine.

Preventing release of drug in the stomach may be useful from two viewpoints. First, it protects acid-labile drugs from acid-catalyzed degradation. This phenomenon was already discussed for erythromycin and erythromycin stearate, but it is important for all acid-labile substances. In this case, the drug is protected from endogenous secretions.

The second viewpoint is not to protect the drug from the patient, but rather to protect the patient from the drug. Some drugs are irritating to the stomach and can cause local distress, nausea, and vomiting. Such drug substances include iron salts, diethylstilbestrol, and aspirin to a somewhat lesser extent. Drug release can be delayed until drug reaches the small intestine by using an acid-resistant coating and thus avoiding local toxicity in the stomach. Because release of drug from these types of formulations is clearly dependent on stomach-emptying rate, absorption of drug may be significantly affected by changes in stomach-emptying patterns. Consider the following example.

As will be considered in more detail in the next chapter, food can cause a marked decrease in stomach-emptying rate. Bogentoft et al. (4) compared the effect of food on the absorption efficiency of drug from enteric-coated aspirin tablets and from a formulation of enteric-coated aspirin granules contained in conventional capsules. The results of this study are summarized in Figure 5.2. Plasma salicylate levels (salicylate

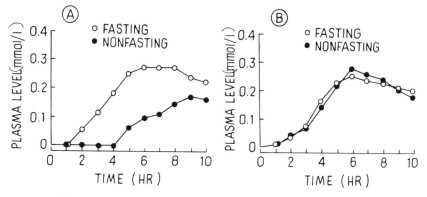

Figure 5.2. Mean plasma salicylate levels in eight subjects following single 1.0-g doses of aspirin as enteric-coated tablets (A) and enteric-coated granules in capsules (B) under fasting and nonfasting conditions. (Reproduced with permission from reference 4. Copyright 1978, Springer-Verlag.)

is the major metabolite formed by hydrolysis of aspirin) from the two formulations are similar under fasting conditions. Food did not affect absorption from the granules but caused a marked delay and reduction in absorption from the coated tablets. Tablets yielded essentially zero absorption for 4 h after dosing, presumably a result of the tablets being retained in the stomach and the acid-resistant coating remaining intact during that period. The lack of effect by food on the encapsulated granules is consistent with the more diffuse nature of this dosage form and the ease that granules may move into the intestine after the capsule has dissolved.

Controlled-Release Formulations

Although the concept of sustained or controlled delivery of orally administered drugs has existed for some time, a remarkable increase in interest in this type of dosage form has arisen during the last decade. Current interest has been due to the simultaneous maturation of various factors including greater appreciation of the advantages of controlled drug release and the development of novel polymer systems and devices that are suitable for controlled delivery of oral dosage forms (5,6).

Some drug substances that are currently available in controlled-release form are listed on page 51. Several commercial products are available for many drugs or drug combinations, and the number of drug substances available in controlled-release form is increasing rapidly.

Most of the oral controlled-release products currently available include diuretic and cardiovascular drugs, respiratory drugs, and compounds acting on the central nervous system. Little attention has been paid to antimicrobial agents. Only one compound, tetracycline, is available in controlled-release form. Controlled release of antimicrobial agents that have appropriate pharmacokinetic properties appears to represent an area of virtually untapped potential. However, this situation may remain so until more information is available regarding the temporal relationships between circulating antibiotic levels and the efficacy of antibacterial effect.

Advantages of Controlled Drug Release. Controlled-release dosage forms are frequently more expensive than conventional formulations and can be justified only when they offer one or more therapeutic advantages. Some of the advantages of controlled-release dosage forms are as follows:

1. rapid onset and maintenance of therapeutic drug levels

2. reduced dosing frequency

3. reduced fluctuations in drug levels

4. reduced total amount of drug used

5. reduced inconvenience to the patient and increased compliance

6. reduced patient care time

7. less nighttime dosing

8. more uniform pharmacological response

9. reduced GI irritation

10. reduced side effects

Although each of these advantages is important from one viewpoint or another, the only advantages relevant to this chapter are items 1, 2, 3, and 8. Item 1 can be achieved only if the controlled-release formulation contains a fast-release component, or if a fast-release formulation is used

Some Substances Available in Controlled-Release Form

Vitamins, Minerals, and Hormones

Ascorbic acid
Iron preparations
Methyltestosterone
Nicotinic acid
Potassium
Pyridoxine
Vitamin combinations

Diuretic and Cardiovascular Drugs

Acetazolamide
Ethaverine HCl
Isosorbide dinitrate
Nicotinyl alcohol
Nitroglycerin
Papaverine HCl
Pentaerythritol tetranitrate
Procainamide
Quinidine gluconate and sulfate
Reserpine

CNS Drugs

Amphetamine sulfate
Aspirin
Caffeine
Chlorpromazine
Dextroamphetamine sulfate
Diazepam
Diethylpropion HCl
Fluphenazine
Indomethacin
Lithium
Meprobamate
Methamphetamine HCl
Orphenadrine citrate
Pentobarbital
Pentylenetetrazole
Perphenazine
Phenmetrazine HCl
Phenobarbital
Phentermine HCl
Phenylpropanolamine HCl
Prochlorperazine

Respiratory Agents

Aminophylline
Brompheniramine maleate
Carbinoxamine maleate
Chlorpheniramine maleate
Combination, antitussive
Combination, expectorant
Combination, upper respiratory
Dexchlorpheniramine maleate
Dimethindene maleate
Diphenylpraline HCl
Dyphylline
Phenylpropanolamine HCl
Pseudoephedrine HCl and sulfate
Theophylline
Trimeprazine
Tripelennamine HCl
Xanthine combinations

Antimicrobial

Tetracycline

Gastrointestinal Drugs

Belladonna alkaloids
Hexocyclium methylsulfate
1-Hyoscyamine sulfate
Isopropamide iodide
Prochlorperazine maleate
Tridihexethyl chloride

Other

Pyridostigmine bromide

SOURCE: Reproduced with permission from reference 5. Copyright 1983, Marcel Dekker.

to initiate therapy. Items 2 and 3 describe the essence of controlled release, which is to obtain prolonged circulating drug levels with less fluctuation compared to conventional dosage forms and to achieve these drug levels with less frequent drug administration. Item 8, which also is a primary goal of controlled-release dosage, may be predicted from theoretical drug level-response relationships but is difficult to prove experimentally.

Disadvantages of Controlled Drug Release. The major potential disadvantages of controlled-release dosage forms are as follows:

- possibility of dose-dumping
- reduced potential for accurate dose adjustment
- slow absorption may delay onset of activity
- increased potential for first-pass metabolism
- possible reduction in systemic availability
- drug release period restricted to residence time in the GI tract.

"Dose-dumping," a term used to describe the inadvertent rapid release of drug material due to faulty formulation or some other factor, is particularly important for potent drugs that have a narrow therapeutic index. However, good manufacturing practice and also the highly sophisticated dosage forms currently appearing on the market reduce the possibility of dose-dumping.

Administering a fraction of a tablet or capsule to achieve capsule fine dose adjustment is more difficult with some controlled-release dosage forms than with others. For example, controlled-release tablets, which are granules in a tablet matrix, can readily be subdivided to obtain a fraction of a dose. On the other hand, formulations such as repeat-action tablets or osmotic pump devices lose their sustained-release properties after the dosage form is fractured. Slow absorption inevitably delays the onset of drug activity from an initial dose, but this delay is probably unimportant with repeated doses. Increased first-pass metabolism may occur for drugs that undergo extensive hepatic clearance, but only if hepatic clearance is saturable following rapid absorption from conventional doses. If saturation does not occur with conventional oral dosages, and if hepatic clearance is first-order in nature, then the same proportion of an oral dose will be cleared during the first pass through the liver regardless of the absorption rate.

Although reduced drug absorption due to first-pass metabolism may be unimportant, at least in the light of present knowledge, reduced and variable absorption from controlled-release drugs from the GI tract due to formulation factors has been documented. This problem is demonstrated in Figures 5.3 and 5.4, which show a wide range in absorption

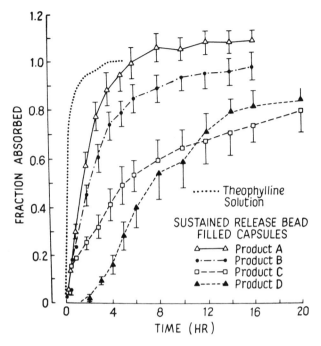

Figure 5.3. Cumulative absorption plots of theophylline from four controlled-release capsules and an aqueous solution. Error bars indicate 1 standard deviation. (Reproduced with permission from reference 7. Copyright 1978, Massachusetts Medical Society.)

rate and efficiency from commercial controlled-release capsules and tablets of theophylline (7). This situation is unacceptable from clinical and regulatory viewpoints, the latter requiring equivalent bioavailability from different sustained-release formulations of the same drug entity.

Residence time within the GI tract is a potential disadvantage associated with oral controlled-release products, and residence time distinguishes oral controlled-release from parenteral controlled-release dosage forms. The actual time period available for an oral dosage form to effectively release drug for absorption is not well established and may vary among individuals. The residence time of the dosage form in the stomach is variable depending on the activity of the patient, the presence of food in the stomach, and direct or indirect interactions with other drugs. After leaving the stomach, the dosage form along with dissolved drug passes into the optimum absorption region of the proximal small intestine. Distal to this region, absorption becomes less efficient, and the drug is furthermore exposed to the bacterial microflora. Because of variable GI transit time and also these other factors, estimating the optimum release period for an oral controlled-release dosage form becomes difficult. Assuming

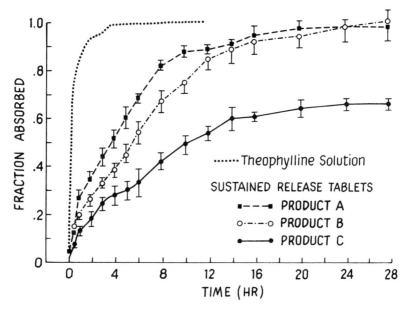

Figure 5.4. Cumulative absorption plots of theophylline from three controlled-release tablets and an aqueous solution. Error bars indicate 1 standard deviation. (Reproduced with permission from reference 7. Copyright 1978, Massachusetts Medical Society.)

that absorption efficiency is constant throughout the entire period that drug is in the GI tract is speculative also.

Drugs That Are Unsuited for Controlled Release. Apart from these disadvantages, some drug types are inherently unsuited for controlled-release formulations. Some typical characteristics are listed here.

- short biological half-life
- long biological half-life
- potent drug with narrow therapeutic index
- large doses
- poorly absorbed

- low or slow solubility
- active absorption
- time course of circulating drug levels does not agree with pharmacological response
- extensive first-pass metabolism.

A controlled-release dosage form for a drug that has a short biological half-life of less than 2 h or is administered in large doses may need to contain a prohibitively large amount of drug. On the other hand, drugs with a long biological half-life of 8 h or more are sufficiently sustained in the body from conventional doses, and prolonged-release forms are generally not necessary.

Absorption of poorly water-soluble compounds is often limited by their dissolution rate. Incorporation of such compounds into a controlled-release formulation is therefore unnecessary and is likely to reduce overall absorption efficiency. Administering drugs such as warfarin, whose pharmacological effect is considerably delayed relative to its blood profile, is of no therapeutic advantage. Similarly, incorporating compounds such as fluorouracil, amino acids, and perhaps some β-lactam antibiotics and thiazide diuretics that appear to exhibit reduced absorption efficiency at sites distal from the proximal small intestine is likely to reduce absorption efficiency while achieving little or no prolongation of effect. As stated previously, if a drug undergoes extensive first-pass hepatic clearance that is saturable with conventional fast-release dosages, then systemic availability may be decreased because of nonsaturation of the clearance mechanisms from a controlled-release dosage form. However, if hepatic clearance is not saturated with conventional doses, then slower absorption of drug should not cause an increase in first-pass presystemic clearance.

Although the preceding lists contain useful general rules on which to base decisions regarding whether to consider a controlled-release dosage form for a particular drug, there are inevitable exceptions to these rules. Nitroglycerin is reported to have a short biological half-life of less than 0.5 h. It is rapidly metabolized by the liver and is generally considered to be poorly absorbed from oral doses. However, a large number of controlled-release oral nitroglycerin products are available, in addition to an increasing number of topical and transdermal preparations. The low circulating levels of nitroglycerin obtained from these products are thought to provide adequate prophylaxis against angina attacks, but would not be adequate to treat an acute angina episode. At the other end of the scale, many of the drugs listed on page 51 have biological half-lives greater than 8 h. Controlled release of these products may reduce toxic side effects simply by preventing the sharp initial peaks in circulating drug levels that may occur with conventional doses. However, these products are unlikely to provide more sustained blood levels or prolonged therapeutic effect compared to conventional dosage forms.

Renewed interest in controlled release has led to a variety of new formulations. Products that are representative of well-established release forms and also some more novel categories are summarized in Table 5.1. This list will undoubtedly increase as more novel dosage forms are introduced. Microencapsulation and osmotic pressure systems are likely to find more applications. Other products that prolong GI residence time by adhesion, for example nitroglycerin (tablets), or by use of low density hydrated gels, for example diazepam, have been introduced. These types of dosage forms may undergo extensive development for other drugs in the future.

Table 5.1—Oral Controlled-Release Dosage Forms

Category	Product	Active Ingredient
Slow erosion with initial fast release dose	Tedral SA	Theophylline, ephedrine HCl, phenobarbital
Erosion core only	Tenuate Dospan	Diethylpropion HCl
Repeat action tablets	Chlor-Trimeton Repetabs	Pseudoephedrine sulfate, chlorpheniramine maleate
Pellets in capsules	Combid Spansule	Isopropamide iodide, prochlorperazine maleate
Pellets in tablets	Theo-Dur	Theophylline
Leaching	Desbutal Gradumet	Methamphetamine HCl, pentobarbital sodium
Ion-exchange resins	Biphetamine	Amphetamine, dextroamphetamine
Complexation	Rynata	Chlorpheniramine, phenylephrine, and pyrilamine tannate
Microencapsulation	Nitrospan	Nitroglycerin
Flotation–diffusion	Valrelease	Diazepam
Osmotic pressure	Acutrim	Phenylpropanolamine

Pharmacokinetics of Controlled Release. Despite the large and ever-expanding array of formulations devoted to oral controlled-release, and despite the complex and varied physical properties involved in the release of drug from these formulations, the number of kinetic models that are necessary to describe overall drug release phenomena from existing dosage forms is relatively small (5). The major release patterns are summarized in simple graphical form in Figure 5.5. The patterns can be divided into two major categories, those that release drug at a slow zero- or first-order rate, and those that provide an initial rapid dose followed by slow zero- or first-order release of the sustained component. The sustained nature of drug release from these dosage forms, even when a fast-release component is present, leads to considerable problems in in vitro dissolution testing. These problems currently are being addressed by official compendia and regulatory agencies.

For conventional oral dosage products, in vitro dissolution criteria are expressed in terms of the fastest possible dissolution rate, that is, there is no upper limit. However, the situation is quite different for controlled-release products. The optimum dissolution rate for controlled-release products is not the fastest rate that can be obtained, but rather some intermediate value that will reflect prolonged release of drug in the

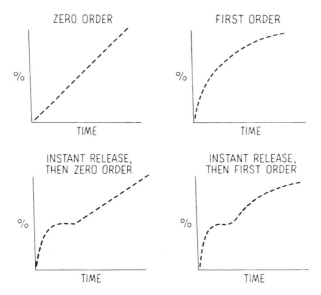

Figure 5.5. In vitro drug release characteristics from oral controlled-release dosage forms.

GI tract. Thus, for these products, a dissolution window is required, and deviation from the optimum rate can be too fast or too slow.

Because of the difficulty of establishing guidelines for these dosage forms, the large number of formulations, and the different release profiles as illustrated in Figure 5.5, no official guidelines for in vitro dissolution tests of oral controlled-release dosage forms exist at the present time. Also, relationships between in vitro drug release and in vivo bioavailability characteristics are not clearly established. The appropriateness of a controlled-release formulation and equivalence between different controlled-release products or between controlled-release and conventional products must currently be based on in vivo data.

Controlled-release dosage forms are entering a new era because of development, and because of more rigid testing and characterization in terms of in vitro–in vivo relationships, predicted and actual release patterns, and pharmacokinetic–pharmacodynamic relationships.

Summary

1. Solution dosages and suspensions generally give rise to more satisfactory bioavailability than capsules or tablets.

2. Coated tablets or capsules may be used to protect the drug from

acid degradation in the stomach, or to prevent local irritation in the stomach.

3. Controlled-release formulations are used to prolong drug activity, reduce fluctuation in blood concentrations, and increase patient convenience and compliance. Controlled-release formulations represent one of the most active areas in the pharmaceutical industry. The potential advantages and disadvantages of controlled release should be considered before initiating a development program for a particular compound.

Literature Cited

1. Welling, P. G.; In *Progress in Drug Metabolism;* Bridges, J. W., Chasseaud, L. F., Eds.; Wiley: New York, Vol. 4, 1980; 131–163.
2. Cadwallader, C. D. *Biopharmaceutics and Drug Interactions;* Hoffmann–LaRoche: Nutley, NJ, 1971.
3. Lindenbaum, J.; Mellow, M. H.; Blackstone, M. O.; Butles, V. P. *New Engl. J. Med.* **1971,** *285,* 1344–1347.
4. Bogentoft, C.; Carlsson, I.; Ekenved, G.; Magnusson, A. *Eur. J. Clin. Pharmacol.* **1978,** *14,* 315–355.
5. Welling, P. G. *Drug Dev. Ind. Pharm.* **1983,** *9,* 1185–1225.
6. *Sustained and Controlled Release Drug Delivery Systems;* Robinson, J. R. , Ed.; Marcel Dekker: New York, 1978.
7. Weinberger, M.; Hendeles, L.; Bighley, L. *New Engl. J. Med.* **1978,** *299,* 852–857.

6

Clinical Factors Affecting Drug Absorption

The efficiency with which an orally administered drug is absorbed and also its absorption rate (i.e., its overall bioavailability) are usually determined in a panel of healthy individuals under controlled and generally fasting conditions in the absence of other drugs. This type of testing procedure is required by regulatory agencies so that drug bioavailability can be established under controlled conditions without interference from other substances.

In clinical practice, however, drugs are seldom taken under such ideal conditions. Patients who are receiving medication may be suffering from a variety of illnesses, particularly those involving the GI tract, that could affect drug absorption. Similarly, patients often receive more than one drug at the same time. This situation is particularly true in hospitals and in geriatric therapy, where it is common practice for patients to receive several drugs simultaneously. Medication may also be taken under varying situations relative to meals. In fact, meal times are often used as reminders for drug dosage. Remembering to take two tablets at breakfast time is easier than taking them at 10 a.m. or 1 h before breakfast. So meal times, from a purely practical point of view, are often convenient but not always the best times to take medication.

These conditions—diseases of the GI tract, drug–drug interactions, and drug–food interactions—are often present in varying degrees, either individually or collectively, when drugs are administered. This chapter

0065-7719/86/0185-0059$06.00/1
© 1986 American Chemical Society

will show that these conditions can cause substantial and often unpredictable changes in drug absorption (1).

The Influence of GI Disease on Drug Absorption

Diseases of the GI tract are potentially important conditions affecting drug absorption. A survey conducted in 1968 showed that digestive diseases were responsible for 10–15% of hospital admissions, 30% of major operations, and 9% of all deaths in the United States (2). The term GI disease is difficult to define because it can include such conditions as diseases of the liver, pancreas, and other organs and tissues closely but indirectly related to the GI tract. Discussion in this chapter is limited to those conditions and surgical procedures directly involving the GI tract, diseases of the stomach, surgery, diseases of the small and large intestine, and intestinal infections.

Diseases of the Stomach. Despite the large number of diseases affecting the stomach, very little is known regarding their influence on drug absorption. Many conditions that might be expected to have a profound effect on drug absorption, for example, carcinoma or peptic stricture, have not been studied.

One condition that has been studied to a small extent and that is currently of interest in some laboratories is achlorhydria, which occurs when diminished secretion of hydrochloric acid results in relatively alkaline stomach contents. The results of the few studies that have been done have not led to an altered drug absorption pattern that would be expected from principles based on pH-dependency of ionization and lipophilicity. Achlorhydria has no apparent effect on the absorption of phenoxymethylpenicillin, but caused an increase in the absorption of aspirin (3,4). Increased absorption of aspirin in this case was presumably due to faster tablet dissolution. Tablet dissolution was favored over drug absorption as an explanation because the increased ratio of ionized to un-ionized drug in the relatively alkaline conditions due to achlorhydria should have decreased, rather than increased, the drug absorption rate. More work needs to be done in this area to determine if the achlorhydric patient is at risk regarding drug absorption, and to establish dosing guidelines if risk is involved.

Surgery. Surgical procedures that involve removal of part of the GI tract might be expected to influence drug absorption as a consequence of reduction in the epithelial surface area or by changes in motility or secretory patterns. Knowing how these procedures actually influence drug absorption would be useful, but again very little information is available. Generating information from these patient populations is notoriously difficult, and the present rate of progress suggests that it may be some time before the relationships between GI surgery, drug absorption, and therapeutic consequences are understood. Some interactions that have been reported for stomach surgery are listed in Table 6.1 (5).

Table 6.1—Effects of Stomach Surgery on Drug Absorption

Procedure	Effect on Drug Absorption		
	Increased	Unchanged	Decreased
Partial gastrectomy	Ethanol p-Aminosalicylate	Ampicillin Digoxin Isoniazid	Cephalexin Ethionamide Folate Iron Nitrofurantoin Sulfamethoxazole
Antrectomy, gastroduodenostomy		Ethambutol Isoniazid Quinidine Sulfisoxazole Tetracycline	
Antrectomy, gastroduodenostomy, vagotomy			Ethambutol Quinidine Sulfisoxazole

Partial gastrectomy has caused reduced absorption of some drugs, but the reduction has been attributed to different factors. For example, reduced iron absorption was attributed to loss of a gastric factor necessary for inorganic iron absorption, and reduced ethionamide absorption was attributed to slow dissolution causing unreliable absorption in postresection patients. Absorption of ethambutol, quinidine, and sulfisoxazole is reduced in cases of gastric surgery with vagotomy, but absorption of these and other compounds is not affected by gastric surgery alone, and this fact suggests that delayed stomach emptying due to loss of vagal control caused the actual reduction in absorption. Mean serum levels of quinidine, ethambutol, and sulfisoxazole in patients before and after gastric surgery with vagotomy are shown in Figure 6.1.

Resection of the small bowel is a surgical procedure commonly done to reduce nutrient absorption in obese individuals. This type of procedure might reasonably be expected to decrease drug absorption. However, as with gastric surgery, a decrease does not necessarily occur. Absorption of hydrochlorothiazide, levonorgestrol, and norethindrone is reduced following intestinal shunt surgery, but absorption of ampicillin, digoxin, phenazone, and propylthiouracil appear to be unaffected.

Loss of sulfasalazine activity for treatment of Crohn's disease following colonic resection is an interesting example of an indirect effect by

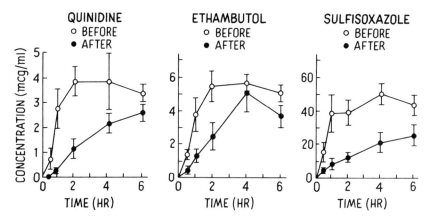

Figure 6.1. Mean serum levels of quinidine, ethambutol, and sulfisoxazole in nine patients before and after antrectomy with gastroduodenostomy and selective vagotomy. (Reproduced with permission from Scand. J. Gastroent. **1975**, 10, 43.)

surgery affecting drug absorption and action. Sulfasalazine is partially absorbed in the intact form into the systemic circulation, but most of the drug is cleaved at the azo linkage by intestinal bacteria to release the active moiety 5-aminosalicylate. Reduced effectiveness of sulfasalazine in postsurgery patients appears to result from loss of colonic bacteria following resection. The effects of intestinal surgery on drug absorption are summarized in Table 6.2 (6).

Table 6.2—Effects of Intestinal Surgery on Drug Absorption

	Effect on Drug Absorption	
Procedure	*Unchanged*	*Decreased*
Intestinal shunt surgery	Ampicillin Digoxin Phenazone Propylthiouracil	Hydrochlorothiazide Levonorgestrol Norethindrone
Colonic resection		Sulfasalazine

Diseases of the Small Intestine. A large number of diseases can afflict the small intestine. Again, information on most of these diseases is fragmentary and provides little substantive insight into their overall effect on drug absorption. However, two conditions, celiac disease and Crohn's disease, have been studied extensively, and reported apparent effects of these conditions on drug absorption are summarized in Table 6.3.

Celiac disease is an inflammatory condition of the proximal small intestine that is caused by ingestion of gluten, which is a viscous protein

Table 6.3—Apparent Effects of Intestinal Diseases on Drug Absorption

	Effect on Drug Absorption		
Condition	Increased	Unchanged	Decreased
Celiac disease	Aspirin Cephalexin Clindamycin Erythromycin Fusidate Propranolol Sulfamethoxazole Trimethoprim	Ampicillin Indomethacin Lincomycin Methyldopa Pivmecillinam Rifampin	Acetaminophen Amoxicillin Penicillin V Pivampicillin Practolol
Crohn's disease	Clindamycin Fusidate Oxprenolol Propranolol Sulfamethoxazole Trimethoprim	Erythromycin Hydrocortisone Rifampin	Acetaminophen Cephalexin Lincomycin Methyldopa Metronidazole

contained in cereals. The condition is generally kept in remission by a gluten-free diet.

Crohn's disease is also an inflammatory condition, but it differs from celiac disease because it tends to occur in the distal small intestine and proximal large intestine, is of largely unknown etiology, and is usually treated with steroids and sulfasalazine, although it may require surgical resection in severe cases.

Both celiac and Crohn's disease cause malabsorption of nutrients, and therefore might be expected to have a similar effect on drug absorption. However, studies conducted in patients have produced a variety of results (7). Both diseases may cause decreased absorption as shown in Table 6.3, but both may also cause increased absorption or be without effect. The underlying mechanisms causing these changes are not understood. Some of the effects are quite dramatic, for example, circulating levels of fusidate, propranolol, and trimethoprim are approximately doubled in celiac patients compared to normal controls.

The unexpected increase in the apparent absorption of some drugs in patients with celiac and Crohn's disease has led to attempts to understand why this increase should occur. For example, increased absorption of propranolol in celiac disease has been attributed to altered drug diffusion from the proximal small intestine, and also to saturable first-pass metabolism. Present evidence seems to favor the latter explanation, but this is not the complete story. One factor that is common to celiac and Crohn's disease is an increased erythrocyte sedimentation rate. This phenomenon occurs in many inflammatory conditions including rheumatoid arthritis. As indicated in Figure 6.2, propranolol levels are

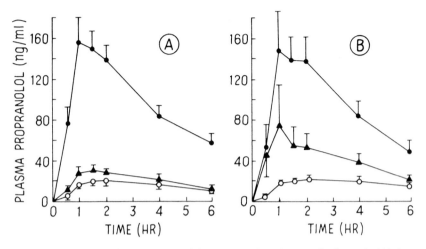

Figure 6.2. Mean plasma propranolol concentrations (± standard error) (A) in healthy controls (○) and in patients with rheumatoid arthritis with ESR ≤ 20 mm/ h (▲) and with ESR > 20 mm/h (●), and (B) in healthy controls (○) and in patients with Crohn's disease with ESR ≤ 20 mm/h (▲) and with ESR > 20 mm/ h (●). (Reproduced with permission from reference 6. Copyright 1979, Macmillan Journals Ltd.)

markedly increased in patients with raised erythrocyte sedimentation rates who are suffering from Crohn's disease, and also from rheumatoid arthritis. The latter condition is unlikely to affect drug absorption so that the increased drug levels may not result entirely from drug absorption effects. Further research has established that erythrocyte sedimentation rates are associated with elevated plasma levels of the acute phase protein α_1-acid glycoprotein (AAG). Propranolol, together with many other basic drugs, binds avidly to this protein so that when levels of AAG increase in conditions of stress, fever, or other inflammatory conditions including celiac and Crohn's disease and rheumatoid arthritis, more of the circulating drug binds to the protein. This binding causes a shift in the distribution of drug from tissue into plasma. Thus, part of the increase in circulating propranolol levels in celiac and Crohn's disease, and possibly other conditions, appears to result from redistribution of drug into the plasma at the expense of tissues as a consequence of increased AAG levels, as well as an absorption effect (8).

Recent studies in rats showed that adjuvant-induced arthritis can cause a threefold increase in circulating propranolol levels compared to normal controls after intravenous injection where no absorption is involved (9).

Diseases of the Large Intestine. Diseases of the large intestine are less likely to affect drug absorption than those in the small intestine because most absorption is complete by the time drug has reached this distal region of the GI tract. However, diseases of the large intestine are a potential problem for drugs that are absorbed distally, particularly from controlled-release formulations. As with most other regions of the GI tract, the influence of diseases of the large intestine on drug absorption is largely unknown.

Loss of sulfasalazine activity for the treatment of Crohn's disease following colonic resection was previously described. Loss of activity in that instance is due largely to loss of bacterial flora following surgery, thereby preventing cleavage of the molecule to release 5-aminosalicylate. Another study reported no alteration in hydrocortisone absorption in patients who have regional enteritis and active ulcerative colitis. The problem of large bowel disease appears not to have been addressed for rectal administration where varying proportions of administered drug may be absorbed from the colon and distal large intestine.

Intestinal Infections. The GI tract is susceptible to a variety of infections such as shigellosis, gastroenteritis, cholera, food poisoning, and infestations by worms and protozoa. Although these conditions present their own particular problems for the patient and call for prompt treatment, the main problem as far as drug absorption is concerned is that intestinal infections frequently cause diarrhea, which can affect drug absorption. This effect has been demonstrated for ampicillin and nalidixic acid. The absorption of both compounds was reduced in children with acute shigellosis, and the extent of reduction in absorption was related to the severity of the condition. Pregnancies have occurred after the use of oral contraceptives during periods of diarrhea. Poor GI absorption was presumably due to rapid transit of the contraceptive pill.

Drug–Drug Interactions Affecting Absorption

Drug–drug interactions leading to improved or impaired absorption of one or both of the interacting substances is a major problem in therapy, particularly in severely ill or geriatric patients who may have to take several oral medications simultaneously. Some compounds that have been shown to affect the absorption of other drugs will be discussed in the next two sections. Many interactions have been reported in detail (10). Interactions that have been reported can be conveniently divided into indirect action and direct action.

Indirect Action. One of the primary factors affecting drug absorption is stomach-emptying rate. Any drug that can alter this rate is likely to influence the absorption of other drugs or itself (11).

Propantheline is a drug with anticholinergic activity. It reduces GI motility, stomach-emptying rate, and gastric acid secretion. It is used as adjuvant therapy for treatment of peptic ulcer. Metoclopramide, on the other hand, increases stomach-emptying rate and is used to prevent gastric reflux. These two agents have marked and opposite effects on the absorption of other drugs, presumably because of their opposing influences on stomach-emptying rate. Typically, metoclopramide increases the absorption rates of such drugs as acetaminophen, ethanol, levodopa, and lithium; propantheline decreases the absorption rate of acetaminophen, ethanol, lithium, and hydrochlorothiazide. Although these results suggest the possibility of the rarest and most elusive of all goals, a general rule regarding drug absorption, exceptions to the rule have already been reported from our laboratory and elsewhere. Specifically, the absorption of chlorothiazide, and also digoxin from a particular brand of tablets, has been reported to be increased by propantheline and reduced by metoclopramide.

Increased absorption efficiency of both chlorothiazide and digoxin in the presence of propantheline, and the opposite effect with metoclopramide, is probably due to dissolution rate-limited absorption. Slower stomach emptying permits a greater percentage of the drug to pass into solution before it passes into the small intestine. An alternative explanation involving saturable and site-specific absorption has been proposed for chlorothiazide, but this explanation has yet to be confirmed.

Neomycin is administered orally for bowel sterilization and also for treatment of enterocolitis. In addition to its antibiotic effect, neomycin also has a variety of effects on the GI tract including binding and precipitation of bile acids and fatty acids, interference with the micellar phase, and consequent inhibition of fat absorption. In addition to its effects on fat absorption, neomycin also impairs absorption of vitamin A, vitamin B_{12}, digoxin, and penicillin V.

Direct Action. Antacids, kaolin-pectin, charcoal, cholestyramine, and metal ions exert their effects on other drugs directly. By far the most common among these agents are the antacids. These substances, which are taken in large quantities by many people, can interact with other drugs or other dosage forms in several ways that lead usually to reduced drug absorption. By raising the gastrointestinal pH, antacid preparations may increase the solubility of acids, but decrease the solubility of bases. Antacids may also increase the degree of ionization of acids and decrease that of bases. The solubility effect should favor the absorption of acids, but the ionization effect should favor that of bases. Antacids that contain heavy metal ions may also chelate with other drugs.

Regardless of the mechanism or mechanisms involved, absorption of most drugs is reduced by antacids. For example, the absorption of digoxin, isoniazid, penicillamine, most tetracyclines, chlorpromazine, and vitamin A is reduced in the presence of antacid preparations. Most of these interactions have resulted in marked reduction in absorption, ranging from 10–45% for chlorpromazine to 80% for some tetracyclines. The effect of sodium bicarbonate on tetracycline absorption is illustrated in Figure 6.3 (12).

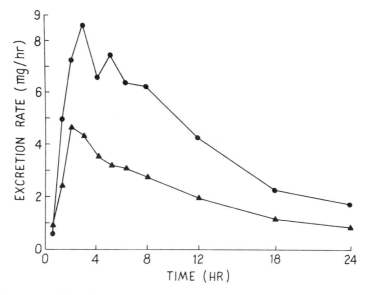

Figure 6.3. Effect of sodium bicarbonate on tetracycline HCl absorption. Mean urinary excretion rates in subjects receiving a single 250-mg tetracycline HCl capsule with 200 mL of water (●) or with 200 mL of water containing 2 g of sodium bicarbonate (▲). (Reproduced with permission from reference 12. Copyright 1971, C. V. Mosby.)

Interestingly, increased gastric pH due to antacids has caused a marked increase in the absorption of aspirin from an enteric-coated tablet. Although this increase appears to be the only reported interaction of this type, absorption of most drugs from enteric-coated formulations should be accelerated by antacids because of faster dissolution of the acid-resistant, but alkaline-sensitive, enteric coat.

Three other substances, kaolin–pectin, charcoal, and cholestyramine resin, inhibit absorption of other drugs by adsorbing compounds to their surface. Interest in activated charcoal has increased recently because this material not only reduces drug absorption but also increases the elimination rate of substances by trapping them after diffusion or excretion into the GI tract. This method is potentially useful for treatment of drug overdose and poisoning. Increased elimination of phenobarbital, carbamazepine, and phenylbutazone in the presence of GI charcoal is demonstrated in Figure 6.4 (13). A spectacular effect occurs with phenobar-

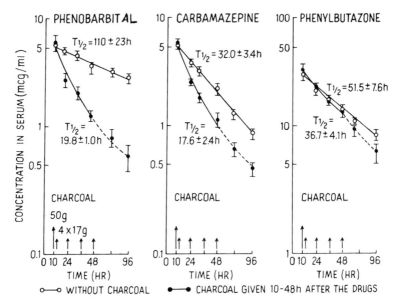

Figure 6.4. Effect of activated charcoal given in multiple doses between 10 and 48 h after the drugs (charcoal doses indicated by arrows) on the elimination rates of phenobarbital, carbamazepine, and phenylbutazone. Half-lives were calculated from concentrations at 10, 24, 32 and 48 h, mean ± standard error in five volunteers. (Reproduced with permission from reference 13. Copyright 1980, Springer-Verlag, New York.)

bital, whose elimination half-life was decreased from 110 h to 20 h by charcoal treatment.

Metal ions interact with other drugs by chelation and can substantially reduce drug absorption. Dramatic reduction in serum levels of four different tetracyclines by moderate doses of ferrous sulfate is shown in Figure 6.5 (14). These types of interactions have been recognized for some time, and tetracycline and iron salts should not be administered together. More recently, iron tablets have been shown to inhibit penicillamine absorption (penicillamine is a potent metal chelator) by 75% and also to significantly decrease penicillamine-induced urinary excretion of copper (15). The clinical significance of this study is uncertain, but it is likely to be important because of the magnitude of the effect.

Food–Drug Interactions

As indicated previously, drugs are frequently taken with food, and patients often use mealtimes as reminders to take their medication. However, food can have a marked effect on drug absorption, the degree of interaction, and the direction interaction takes, inhibitory or otherwise,

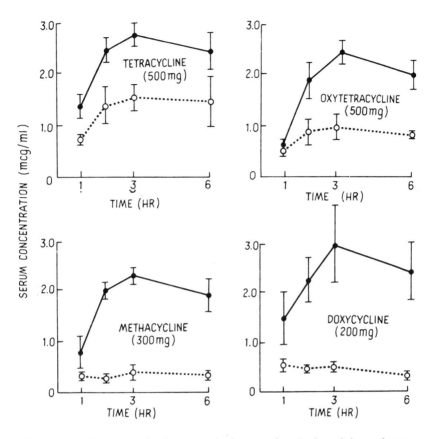

Figure 6.5. Mean serum levels (± standard error) after single oral doses of tetra-cycline, oxytetracycline, methacycline, and doxycycline taken alone (●) or simul-taneously with 200 mg of ferrous sulfate (40 mg of Fe²⁺) (○). (Reproduced with permission from reference 14. Copyright 1970, British Medical Association.)

depending on the drug and the formulation. Generally, the greatest effect is observed when drug is taken immediately after a meal, and the degree of interaction decreases as the time between eating and drug dosing increases. If the drug is taken immediately before a meal, a similar effect is often, but not always, observed to that when it is taken immediately after a meal.

When food is ingested, stomach emptying is delayed, and intestinal motility and GI secretions tend to increase. Splanchnic blood flow also increases, and the degree of increase depends on the type of food. Apart from its action on the GI tract, food also acts as a physical adsorbant and barrier to drug absorption. Substances such as heavy metal ions in food can interact with drugs directly. Considering all of these factors, one might predict that food would reduce or delay drug absorption. This prediction holds true for many drugs and drug formulations, but not universally so. Space does not permit a detailed description of all drug–food interactions. More details on this subject are found in other reviews (15,16).

Some reported drug–food interactions are contained in the list below. Drug absorption can be reduced, delayed, increased, or unaffected by food. Each column in the list contains a variety of drug types including acids, bases, and neutral compounds that have various physical and chemical characteristics. The magnitude of the effects also varies, so that changes in circulating drug concentrations due to food may or may not be clinically important. Some drugs appear in more than one category; for example, aspirin absorption may be both reduced and delayed by food.

Effect of Food on Absorption of Some Drugs

Reduced	Delayed	Unaffected	Increased
Ampicillin	Acetaminophen	Bendroflumethiazide	Alafosfalin
Aspirin	Aspirin	Bevantolol	Carbamazepine
Atenolol	Cephalosporins	Chlorpropamide	Chlorothiazide
Captopril	Sulfonamides	Ethambutol	Diazepam
Ethanol	Diclofenac	Hydralazine	Dicoumarol
Hydrochlorothiazide	Digoxin	Oxazepam	Diftalone
Penicillins (most)	Furosemide	Oxprenolol	Griseofulvin
Tetracyclines (most)	Indoprofen	Phenazone	Labetalol
Iron	Tolmesoxide	Pivampicillin	Metoprolol
Levodopa	Valproate	Propoxyphene	Propranolol
Penicillamine		Tolbutamide	Nitrofurantoin
Sotalol		Tranexamic acid	α-Tocopheryl
Warfarin			nicotinate

The absorption of most penicillins and tetracyclines is reduced by food as are the antihypertensive agents atenolol, sotalol, and hydrochlorothiazide. A recent study showed that penicillamine absorption is markedly reduced not only by food but also, as mentioned earlier, by antacids and ferrous ion (17). These results are not surprising considering the instability of penicillamine in solution and its powerful chelating properties. The reduction in circulating penicillamine levels after oral doses due to food, antacid, and an iron salt is shown in Figure 6.6.

The absorption of several compounds, although not being reduced by food in terms of the total quantity of drug absorbed, is delayed by food. One could argue that this delay is not important because the same quantity of drug ultimately reaches the circulation, but this argument may not be true. Circulating levels of cephradine in fasted and nonfasted

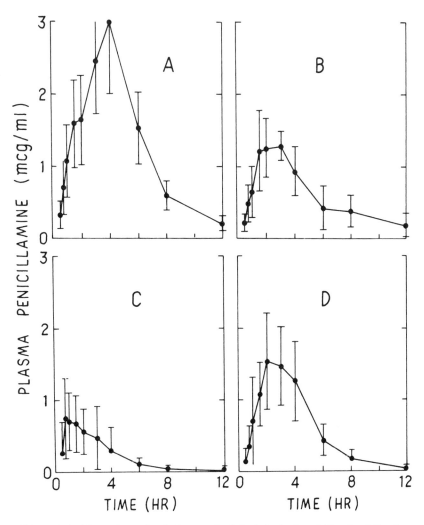

Figure 6.6. *Mean plasma levels (± standard deviation) of penicillamine following single 500-mg oral doses (A) after overnight fast, (B) immediately following a meal, (C) with 300 mg of ferrous sulfate, and (D) with 30 mL of an antacid mixture. (Reproduced with permission from reference 17. Copyright 1983, C. V. Mosby.)*

subjects are shown in Figure 6.7 (*18*). Much lower profiles obtained in nonfasted individuals may be subtherapeutic for less sensitive organisms, but may provide more prolonged activity against more sensitive organisms. Similar results to these have been observed with the oral cephalosporins cephalexin and cefaclor.

Delayed availability has been demonstrated for several new thera-

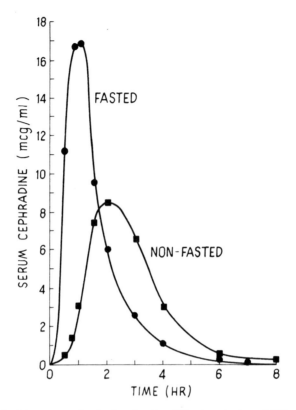

Figure 6.7. *Mean serum levels of cephradine following single oral 500-mg doses of cephradine in capsules to fasted and nonfasted subjects. (Reproduced with permission from reference 18. Copyright 1974, Hall Associates.)*

peutic agents including the anti-inflammatory compounds diclofenac and piroxicam, the antibacterial agent cinoxacin, the hypotensive tolmesoxide, and the antiepileptic valproic acid. Slow absorption in the case of tolmesoxide may be advantageous in reducing the incidence of side effects, and slow absorption of valproic acid may be used to reduce the degree of fluctuation in blood levels and provide more uniform circulating drug levels.

The absorption of some compounds is either unaffected or affected to a small extent by food. The drugs cited are often formulated in solutions or suspensions that are generally less sensitive to food-induced alteration to gastric emptying, but this is not always so. Among the β-blocking agents, the absorption of atenolol and sotalol is decreased by food, bevantolol and oxprenolol are not affected, and absorption of metoprolol, labetalol, and propranolol is increased.

The last column in the list on page 70 describes some drugs whose absorption is increased by food. This column contains the three β-block-ing agents that were just discussed, and circulating levels of metoprolol and propranolol dosed under fasting and nonfasting conditions are shown in Figure 6.8 (*19*).

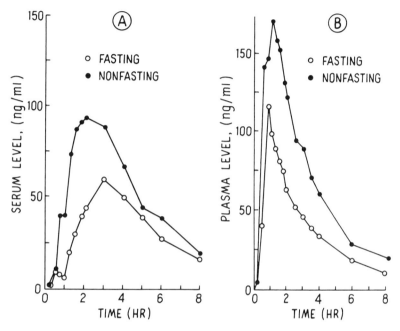

Figure 6.8. Levels of (A) propranolol in serum and (B) metoprolol in plasma in two subjects following single oral doses of 80 mg of propranolol or 100 mg of metoprolol under fasting and nonfasting conditions. (Reproduced with permission from reference 19. Copyright 1977, C. V. Mosby Company.)

Increased drug availability in the presence of food may be rational-ized in terms of increased GI secretions improving compound solubility, or delayed gastric emptying permitting more compound to dissolve by the time it enters the small intestine. However, more specific mechanisms have been proposed for some drugs. Some of the interactions in the list on page 70 are well documented, for example, griseofulvin, pivampi-cillin, and nitrofurantoin. Other interactions have only recently been reported. Increased absorption of the highly metabolized agents meto-prolol, labetalol, and propranolol in the presence of food may be due to increased splanchnic blood flow causing reduced first-pass hepatic clear-ance.

Food-induced increases in drug availability in other recent studies have ranged from moderate effects, as with phenytoin, whose absorption was increased by approximately 27% in nonfasting individuals, to dramatic increases, as in the case of proquazone, mebendazole, and α-tocopheryl nicotinate. Administering the nonsteroidal anti-inflammatory agent proquazone immediately after a meal caused a 2.5-fold increase in peak plasma levels and a twofold increase in areas under 0–24-h plasma curves. However, the most spectacular increase in drug absorption in the presence of food was demonstrated for the peripheral vasodilator, dl-α-tocopheryl nicotinate. The mean peak plasma level and area under the plasma curve were increased 32-fold and 29-fold, respectively, when this vasodilator was given to human volunteers after a standard breakfast, compared to humans in the fasting state. dl-α-Tocopheryl nicotinate appears to be absorbed from the GI tract mainly via the lymphatic system. Marked increase in absorption after food intake may therefore be due to induced flow of bile and pancreatic juices that are necessary for mixed micelle formation, and also to biosynthesis of chylomicrons in the epithelial cells of the GI tract. Both explanations lead to greater lymphatic uptake.

The influence by food on the availability of erythromycin, its stearate salt, and its esters from various products is interesting, and quite confusing. The absorption of erythromycin base and its stearate salt is decreased when administered after a meal, and absorption of erythromycin stearate is inhibited when it is taken with a reduced quantity of water. Repeated-dose studies have shown that enteric-coated erythromycin base is affected less by food than by other film-coated formulations. The esters of erythromycin are less water-soluble and more resistant to acid-catalyzed degradation than the free base or its salts. Therefore, erythromycin esters are likely to be less susceptible to changes in gastric motility or GI secretions after food intake. Consistent with this idea, most studies have reported either unchanged or increased availability of erythromycin estolate and erythromycin ethylsuccinate after postprandial doses. This result is true for all dosage forms of these compounds, including suspensions.

Thus, food ingestion can cause drug absorption to be decreased, increased, delayed, or unaffected. Which of these results occurs depends not only on the drug, but also on the dosage form, the type of food, and on the time interval between eating and dosing. Some drug products including most tetracyclines, penicillins, erythromycin, and perhaps the oral cephalosporins should be taken on an empty stomach. Others, including chlorothiazide, nitrofurantoin, propranolol, proquazone, dl-α-tocopheryl nicotinate, and the esters of erythromycin are more efficiently absorbed when taken after meals. For some drugs, for example chlorpropamide and ethambutol, medication time is not important, at least from an availability viewpoint, when the drug is taken with respect to meals.

Along with disease states and drug–drug interactions, generating simple guidelines regarding drug dosage relative to food is not possible. Each column in the list on page 70 contains a variety of drug products that have various physical and chemical characteristics. However, because the majority of drugs studied are adversely affected or not influenced by food, giving drugs on an empty stomach appears reasonable unless GI irritation or other factors demand otherwise.

Summary

1. Disease states have been shown to alter drug absorption, but information on this subject is fragmentary. Predicting the effect of a particular condition on drug absorption is not possible from current information in most cases. Considering possible changes in drug protein binding and distribution states is important when examining disease-state pharmacokinetics.

2. Many drugs interact in the GI tract to affect absorption. These interactions may be direct or indirect. The direction of change is largely predictable, but there are sufficient exceptions for drugs to be considered individually.

3. Food substances can interact with drugs and lead to reduced, delayed, or increased drug absorption. The extent of interaction, again only partially predictable, may be therapeutically important.

Literature Cited

1. Welling, P. G. In *Progress in Drug Metabolism,* Vol. 4; Bridges, J. W.; Chasseaud, L. F.; Eds.; Wiley: New York, 1980, pp 131–162.
2. Bank, S.; Saunders, S. J.; Marks, I. N.; Novis, B. H.; Barbezat, G. O. In *Drug Treatment Principles and Practice of Clinical Pharmacology and Therapeutics.* Avery, G. S., Ed. ADIS: Sydney Australia, 1980, pp 193–194.
3. Davies, J. A.; Holt, J. M.; Mullinger, B. J. *Antimicrob. Chemother.* **1975,** 1 (Suppl.), 69–70.
4. Pottage, A.; Nimmo, J.; Prescott, L. F.; *J. Pharm. Pharmacol.* **1974,** 26, 144–145.
5. Welling, P. G. In *Pharmacokinetic Basis for Drug Treatment.* Benet, L. Z. et al., Eds.; Raven: New York, 1984, pp 29–47.
6. Welling, P. G.; Tse, Fl. L. S.; *J. Clin. Hosp. Pharm.* **1984,** 9, 163–179.
7. Parsons, R. L.; Hossack, G.; Paddock, G.; *J. Antimicrob. Chemother.* **1975,** 1, 39–50.
8. Schneider, R. E.; Bishop, H.; Hawkins, C. F.; *Brit. J. Clin. Pharmacol.* **1979,** 8, 43–47.
9. Bishop, H.; Schneider, R. E.; Welling, P. G. *Biopharm. Drug Dispos.* **1981,** 2, 291–297.
10. Welling, P. G. *Clin. Pharmacokin.* **1984,** 9, 404–434.
11. Nimmo, W. S.; *Clin. Pharmacokin.* **1976,** 1, 189–208.
12. Barr, W. H.; Adir, J.; Garrettson, L. *Clin. Pharm. Ther.* **1971,** 12, 779–784.
13. Neuvonen, P. J.; Elonen, E. *Eur. J. Clin. Pharmacol.* **1980,** 17, 51–57.
14. Neuvonen, P. J.; Gothini, G.; Hackman, R.; Bjorksten, K. *Brit. Med. J.* **1970,** 4, 532–534.

15. Welling, P. G. *J. Pharmacokin. Biopharm.* **1977,** *5*, 291–334.
16. Toothaker, R. D.; Welling, P. G. *Ann. Rev. Pharmacol.* **1980,** *20*, 173–199.
17. Osman, M. A.; Patel, R. B.; Schuna, A.; Sundstrom, W. R.; Welling, P. G. *Clin. Pharm. Ther.* **1983,** *33*, 465–470.
18. Mischler, T. W.; Sugerman, A. A.; Willard, D. A.; Brannick, L. J.; Neiss, E. S. *J. Clin. Pharmacol.* **1974,** *14*, 604–611.
19. Melander, A.; Danielson, K.; Schersten, B.; Wahlin, E. *Clin. Pharmacol. Ther.* **1977,** *22*, 108–112.

7

Drug Distribution

General Distribution

After entering the general circulation, a drug is carried around the body and distributes to various tissues. The rate and extent to which drug penetrates tissues are influenced by the rate of delivery to the tissues by the circulation, the ease with which it can leave the circulation and enter the tissues, and the affinity of drug for particular tissues (1).

Before considering the various aspects of drug distribution in detail, familiarity with some body fluid volumes would be useful. Table 7.1 presents some average values of some body fluid volumes; considerable variation occurs among individuals. While in the circulation, a drug is contained in a volume of approximately 5 L, or 7% body weight. If a drug distributes into extracellular water, but has difficulty crossing cell membranes to reach intracellular water, then the drug will be contained in a volume of about 15 L, or 21% of body weight. On the other hand, if the drug can penetrate also into intracellular water, then the drug will be contained in a volume of approximately 42 L, or 60% of body weight. Calculation would be simplified if these were the only distribution options open to a drug. In fact, distribution is far more complex. But these simple examples illustrate the effect drug distribution may have on plasma (or serum) drug levels.

Before discussing drug distribution further, plasma and serum should be differentiated. If a blood sample is obtained in the absence of an anticoagulant, the clear supernate recovered after the red cells have been allowed to clot is serum. On the other hand, if a blood sample is obtained

0065–7719/86/0185–0077$07.50/1
© 1986 American Chemical Society

Table 7.1—Volumes of Some Body Fluids

Fluid	Volume (L)	Percent of Body Weight
Plasma	3	4
Blood	5	7
Lymph	10	14
Intracellular water	27	39
Extracellular water	15	21
Total body water	42	60

NOTE: Volume values are approximate for a 70-kg male person.

with an anticoagulant, then the clear supernate recovered after the red cells have been centrifuged is plasma. Thus, plasma differs from serum in that plasma still contains the coagulating factors, while serum has lost these during the coagulation process. From a pharmacokinetic viewpoint, the two fluids can generally be regarded as identical.

Suppose a single bolus intravenous dose of 100 mg of three different drugs was administered to normal individuals, and that the drugs distribute into whole blood, extracellular water, or total body water; these fluids represent volumes of 5, 15, and 42 L, respectively. Suppose also that the drugs distribute homogeneously into these volumes, and that plasma concentrations of unchanged drug can be determined before any significant elimination has occurred. What plasma concentrations would be obtained?

When the 100 mg of drug is in whole blood, and provided the drug equilibrates freely between red cells and plasma, then the drug concentration in plasma is 20 mg/L, or 20 μg/mL. Similarly, when the drug distributes into extracellular water, the drug concentration in plasma is 6.7 μg/mL; when drug distributes into total body water, drug concentration is 2.4 μg/mL.

Therefore, the same quantity of the three different drugs will yield plasma concentrations of 20, 6.7, and 2.4 μg/mL, depending on distribution characteristics. This represents an eightfold range in plasma concentrations for the same quantity of drug.

This example shows that drug distribution can have a marked influence on plasma levels, but unless the distribution characteristics of a drug are known, some false conclusions can be made regarding drug absorption from plasma data alone. In the previous example, one might naively assume that the drug that distributes into extracellular water is absorbed three times more efficiently from an oral dose compared to the drug that distributes into total body water. In fact, both drugs are absorbed to the same extent.

The actual distribution of a drug may be more complex than shown in the previous example. Many drugs bind to plasma proteins, and this binding prevents them from leaving the plasma volume. Drugs may concentrate in red blood cells or may not enter these cells very efficiently; therefore, the blood concentration would differ from the plasma concentration. An example of a drug that concentrates in red cells is the anticancer agent, tubercidin. Approximately 80–98% of this drug concentrates in red cells when added to whole blood (2).

Drugs may have high affinity for particular organs and tissues, particularly fatty tissues, so that the "apparent" distribution volume of the drug may be larger than total body volume. Pentothal is a fat-soluble drug and rapidly enters the brain after it is administered. Subsequently, this drug partially redistributes into body fat and is then slowly released into the general circulation. The initial rapid concentration in brain tissues causes very rapid onset of action; redistribution into fatty tissue causes short duration of action. Digoxin is another drug that is extensively taken up by extravascular tissues; apparent distribution volume is about 500 L, or seven times larger than total body volume. This large apparent distribution volume is not possible if distribution is homogeneous and the drug is clearly concentrated in, or being sequestered by, particular organs and tissues.

Capillary Permeability

To pass from intravascular to extravascular fluids, that is, to leave the general circulation, drugs must cross the capillary membrane. These membranes are "normal" in that they are more permeable to lipophilic than hydrophilic compounds, but are "abnormal" in that they are more permeable to most other compounds than other membranes are (3). Fat-soluble substances tend to cross the capillary membrane rapidly. The anesthetic gases cross essentially as if there was no membrane at all, and very rapid exchange results. Water-soluble molecules cross the membrane more slowly and at a rate that is inversely proportional to molecular size. This permeability is demonstrated in Table 7.2. Small molecules appear to pass through the capillary walls by simple diffusion, whereas large molecules have difficulty getting across. The very slow membrane permeability of albumin is important for drugs that are bound to this macromolecule.

The permeability of capillary membranes is increased or decreased in particular regions of the body to suit their particular purposes. For example, permeability is greatly increased in renal capillaries by pores in the membranes of the renal endothelial cells. Membrane permeability is also increased in the liver by the lack of a complete membrane lining in specialized hepatic capillaries, known as sinusoids. Both factors—porous membranes and lack of membrane lining—facilitate easy and rapid transfer of substances into vital organs of elimination and metabolism.

Table 7.2—Permeability of Muscle Capillary to Water-Soluble Molecules

Molecule	Molecular Weight	Diffusion Coefficient Across Capillary Membrane $(cm^3/s \cdot 100\ g)$
Water	18	3.7
Urea	60	1.8
Glucose	180	0.64
Raffinose	594	0.24
Inulin	5,500	0.036
Myoglobin	17,000	0.005
Serum albumin	69,000	<0.001

SOURCE: Adapted with permission from reference 3.

Perfusion and Diffusion Effects

Distribution of a drug between blood and tissue may be perfusion or diffusion *rate limited*. The distribution of most lipid-soluble drugs is *perfusion rate limited*, that is, transfer between blood and tissue depends upon how fast a particular tissue is perfused by blood. On the other hand, distribution of most water-soluble substances is *diffusion rate limited*, that is, controlled by the rate at which the molecules can diffuse across the membrane.

The rates at which blood perfuses some tissues are shown in Table 7.3 (4). These rates vary enormously, from 10 mL/min · g of lung to only 0.03 mL/min · g of resting muscle or fat. The rate at which a drug is presented to tissue can be described by Equation 7.1.

$$\text{rate} = QC_A \qquad (7.1)$$

where Q is blood flow rate and C_A is the arterial drug concentration entering the tissue. If some drug is taken up by tissue, then the concen-

Table 7.3—Blood Perfusion Rates in Certain Tissues

Tissue	Blood Perfusion Rate $(mL/min \cdot g\ of\ tissue)$
Lung	10
Kidney	4
Thyroid gland	2.4
Adrenal gland	1.2
Liver	0.8
Heart	0.6
Brain	0.5
Muscle	0.03
Fat	0.03

SOURCE: Adapted with permission from reference 4.

tration of drug in venous blood leaving the tissue is C_V, and net tissue uptake is described by Equation 7.2.

$$\text{net rate} = Q (C_A - C_V) \tag{7.2}$$

The tissue–blood distribution ratio can be described by a constant K_p, so that when equilibrium between drug in tissue and arterial blood is reached (if equilibrium is reached), then the amount of drug in tissue is given by Equation 7.3.

$$\text{amount of drug in tissue} = K_p V_T C_A \tag{7.3}$$

where V_T is the tissue volume. Although Equation 7.3 indicates how much drug gets into tissue, a description of how quickly drug gets to the tissue is lacking. This time can be determined if the rate of tissue perfusion is known, and if the distribution is perfusion rate limited. This rate is determined simply by dividing the amount of drug that is in the tissue when equilibrium is reached (Eq. 7.3) by the rate at which drug is introduced to the tissue (Eq. 7.1), as in Equation 7.4. Therefore, the time of tissue uptake depends on the distribution ratio K_p and the perfusion rate to that tissue Q/V_T.

$$
\begin{aligned}
\text{time taken for equilibration} &= K_p V_T C_A / Q C_A \\
&= K_p V_T / Q = K_p / (Q / V_T)
\end{aligned} \tag{7.4}
$$

Consider how Equation 7.4 works for distribution of a fat-soluble drug into the kidney, liver, muscle, and fat. Actual perfusion rates and hypothetical distribution ratios have been given for a drug in Table 7.4 (4). The results obtained in the table show that the time taken for drug to equilibrate in kidney from a constant blood concentration is 0.25 min, whereas equilibration for liver would take 1.25 min, for muscle 33 min, and for fat 1,666.7 min, or nearly 28 h. The longer time taken for drug to equilibrate into those tissues where drug tends to concentrate is simply

Table 7.4—Time Required for Perfusion Rate Limited Drug to Equilibrate in Tissue

Tissue	Perfusion Rate (Q/V_T) (mL/min · mg of tissue)	K_p	Time to Equilibrate $K_p/(Q/V_T)$ (min)
Kidney	4	1	0.25
Liver	0.8	1	1.25
Muscle	0.03	1	33.3
Fat	0.03	50	1,666.7

SOURCE: Adapted with permission from reference 4.

due to the longer perfusion process needed to introduce the required amount of drug to that tissue. An example of a drug of this type is thiopental (pentothal). This lipophilic drug has high affinity for both brain and fat tissue. Because the brain is perfused approximately 16 times faster than fat tissue, drug levels in the brain increase faster. Fat tissue accumulates the drug more slowly because of slower perfusion, but eventually causes redistribution of drug from brain to fat. Eventually, the pentothal levels in brain and fat may be equal, but the largest proportion of the body load is in general fat because of its greater overall mass.

Perfusion-limited drug transport assumes that drug diffusion between blood and tissues is fast. However, this assumption is not always the case, and diffusion may be rate-limiting. Diffusion-limited transport is more common with polar than nonpolar compounds. The best examples of diffusion-limited transport are provided by drug entry into the central nervous system. However, the penetration of many drugs into other tissues is also diffusion rate limited. Drugs enter the prostate gland slowly, and adequate levels of antibiotics are difficult to obtain in this organ. Conversely, avid uptake of environmental contaminants such as pesticide residues into fat tissue is due to the lack of a diffusion barrier for these fat-soluble compounds into fatty tissue (4).

The arguments developed so far in this chapter are based on the equilibrium concept. In many cases however, circulating drug levels are not constant but rise and fall with each dose. In these situations, equilibrium between blood and tissue may not be reached. For example, many antibiotics have short biological half-lives, and maintaining blood levels for sufficient time for therapeutic levels to be achieved in tissues is often difficult.

Binding of Drugs to Plasma Proteins

Many drugs bind to plasma proteins. The most important protein as far as drug binding is concerned is albumin, although binding to other proteins, particularly the orosomucoid α_1-acid-glycoprotein (AAG), may also occur.

Although basic drugs often bind to AAG, acidic drugs bind predominantly to albumin. Albumin is a water-soluble protein with a molecular weight of 69,000. It exists at a concentration of 4 g/100 mL in blood plasma, but exists also at lower concentrations in extravascular fluids. Albumin carries about 100 negative and 100 positive charges and has an isoelectric point of about pH 5. Thus, at a plasma pH of 7.4, albumin has a net negative charge, but nonetheless attracts both anions and cations. The binding of drugs to albumin is usually rapidly reversible. The extent to which a drug binds depends upon the affinity of the drug to albumin, the number of binding sites on the albumin molecule for that particular drug, and the concentrations of both drug and albumin.

Because protein crosses the capillary membrane very slowly, drugs bound to plasma proteins are essentially confined to the same volume as the plasma protein, which is about 3 L. Drugs also bind to extravascular macromolecules, and this binding will be considered later in this chapter. Intravascular binding means that protein-bound drugs cannot reach their site of action, particularly if the site is in some tissue outside the bloodstream. For example, protein-bound drugs cannot cross the blood–brain barrier. They also generally cannot enter the liver, kidney, or other organs to be excreted, although there are some important exceptions to this rule.

The literature contains many values for the percentage of drug binding to plasma proteins. For example, probenecid is approximately 80% bound. This means that 80% of the concentration of total probenecid circulating in plasma is bound to proteins. Practically all assay methods used to measure drug or metabolite concentrations in plasma measure total (bound and unbound) compound. For example, if the total drug concentration in plasma is 10 μg/mL and the drug is 80% bound to plasma proteins, then the concentration of bound drug is 8 μg/mL and the concentration of free or unbound drug is only 2 μg/mL.

Failure to take this type of protein binding into account can cause major errors when calculating the distribution volume of a drug. For example, suppose 100 mg of a drug is administered by bolus intravenous injection, and that the plasma concentration of total drug determined before a significant quantity of drug has been eliminated is 8 μg/mL. If protein binding were ignored, the distribution volume would be calculated as 100/8, which is 12.5 L. Thus, one might conclude that the drug has poor distribution characteristics, and is unlikely to penetrate significantly into extravascular tissues and fluids.

However, the drug is actually 80% bound to plasma proteins. A conventional drug assay would not have detected this level, but a protein-binding determination by equilibrium dialysis or by ultrafiltration would. If the drug is 80% bound to plasma proteins, and the total concentration is 8 μg/mL, then the bound concentration is 80% of 8, or 6.4 μg/mL. As the plasma albumin to which the drug is bound is confined essentially to the plasma volume of 3 L, then the total quantity of drug that is bound (and therefore not free to leave plasma volume and participate in any type of free drug equilibrium) is obtained by multiplying 6.4 by 3000 to yield 19,200 μg, or 19.2 mg. Because this quantity of drug is bound (albeit reversibly) to protein, the quantity must be subtracted from the 100 mg of total drug in the body. This leaves 80.8 mg of drug unbound to protein, and therefore free to equilibrate between plasma water and other fluids. To find the distribution volume, the quantity 80.8 mg must be divided by the free drug concentration of 1.6 μg/mL, which yields a volume of 50.5 L. This volume is four times greater than the volume calculated from the total drug concentration. This distribution volume is similar to the volume of total body water and suggests that, instead of having restricted distribution, this drug is well distributed into tissues, undoubtedly entering both extracellular and intracellular water.

Unfortunately, the influence of protein binding on drug distribution is not as simple as the preceding calculations imply. The calculations take into account binding in plasma, but not the binding and other phenomena that may occur in extravascular fluids and tissues. Drugs may bind to extravascular proteins and other tissues, and giving rise to heterogeneous distribution results, as previously noted for digoxin. Such binding will tend to pull the drug out of plasma, and thereby reduce drug concentration. Reduced drug concentration implies a larger distribution space than actually exists. A drug may thus be subjected to both intravascular and extravascular binding, these factors having opposite effects on the apparent distribution volume of a drug. These effects will be discussed in detail in the next chapter.

Table 7.5 provides a list of the percentage binding of some drugs to plasma proteins at therapeutic drug concentrations. Binding can vary from 0% to almost 100%.

Table 7.5—Percent Binding of Drugs to Plasma Proteins at Therapeutic Drug Levels

Drug	Percent Bound	Drug	Percent Bound
Diazoxide	99	Methotrexate	45
Dicoumarol	98	Methadone	40
Diazepam	96	Meperidine	40
Digitoxin	95	Phenacetin	30
Prednisone	90	Acetaminophen	25
Phenytoin	87	Ampicillin	25
Rifampin	85	Digoxin	23
Chlorpropamide	80	Cephalexin	22
Pentothal	75	Barbital	10
Carbamazepine	72	Promethazine	8
p-Aminosalicylate	65	Antipyrine	4
Glutethimide	54	Isoniazid	0
Carbenicillin	47		

A more mechanistic viewpoint of protein binding would be to consider the equilibrium between bound and unbound drug to exist as in Equation 7.5 (3).

$$[C] + [P_f] \rightleftharpoons [P_f C] \tag{7.5}$$

where $[C]$ is the free drug concentration and $[P_f]$ is the concentration of free receptors. This equation, after taking into account the number of binding sites on the protein molecule for a particular drug, rearranges to Equation 7.6.

$$([C] [nP - P_fC])/[P_fC] = K \qquad (7.6)$$

where n is the number of binding sites per protein molecule, K is the dissociation constant of drug–protein complex, and $[nP]$ equals the total concentration of receptors $(P_f + P_fC)$. Equation 7.6 then rearranges to give Equation 7.7.

$$(K + [C]) [P_fC] = [nP] [C] \qquad (7.7)$$

However, if the relationship in Equation 7.8 is used,

$$r = [P_f]/[P] = (n[C])/(K + [C]) \qquad (7.8)$$

where r equals the number of moles of drug bound per mole of protein, then Equation 7.9 is obtained.

$$K_r = n[C] - r[C] \qquad (7.9)$$

If both sides of Equation 7.9 are divided by $[C]K$, Equation 7.10 is obtained.

$$r/[C] = n/K - r/K \qquad (7.10)$$

If r is plotted against $[C]$ from Equation 7.8, a hyperbolic curve is obtained, as in Figure 7.1. This figure shows that as the concentration of drug increases, the binding sites on the protein molecules start to fill, and the number of molecules of drug per molecule of protein increases. Finally, at saturation, the value of r becomes a constant equal to the value n, the number of binding sites.

If $r/[C]$ is plotted against r from Equation 7.10, a linear plot is obtained, as in Figure 7.2. This figure is the familiar Scatchard plot, which is also used to obtain the value of n. The Scatchard plot may exhibit more than one linear segment, each relating to a different group of binding sites with common affinities. Sometimes these types of plots are used successfully to characterize a particular drug–protein interaction.

Of more interest to pharmacokineticists is the percentage of drug that is bound, or β. The value of β can be defined in terms of the concentrations of free and bound drug as in Equation 7.11.

$$\beta = [P_fC]/([P_fC] + [C]) = 1/\{1 + ([C]/[P_fC])\} \qquad (7.11)$$

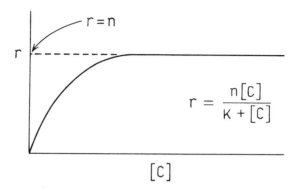

Figure 7.1. Plot of r versus [C] from Equation 7.8.

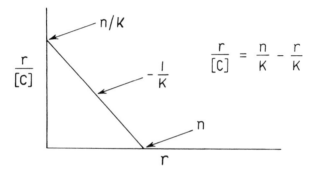

Figure 7.2. Plot of r/[C] versus r from Equation 7.10.

From the relationship in Equation 7.8, the right side of Equation 7.11 rearranges to Equation 7.12.

$$\beta = \frac{1}{1 + K/nP + [C]/nP} \tag{7.12}$$

If β is plotted against $[C]/nP$, or more conveniently against the logarithm of that value, then for different values of K/nP, a series of curves is obtained, as in Figure 7.3. This information shows that at low drug concentrations (the left side of the figure), drugs are maximally bound to protein to an extent dictated by the constant K/nP. As n and P can be considered to be constant for a particular drug, then each of the curves in the figure can be considered to be a function of K. As the drug concentration increases, binding generally becomes saturated so that at very high drug concentrations, free drug is far in excess of bound drug, and the percentage binding, regardless of the value of the binding constant, approaches zero.

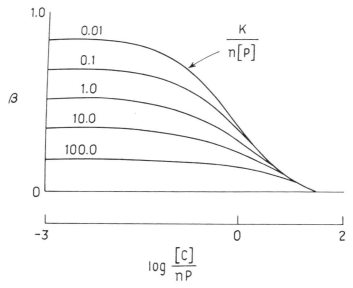

Figure 7.3. Plot of β *versus* log([C]/nP) *from Equation 7.12. (Adapted with permission from reference 3.)*

This figure implies that the percentage binding of drugs continuously changes with changing drug concentrations, so that the binding of a drug will continuously change during a blood concentration profile. Because pharmacokinetic calculations are frequently based on total drug concentrations, a continuously changing relationship between concentrations of bound and unbound drug would be expected. Hence, a continuously changing relationship between the kinetics of total and free drug with changing drug concentrations would also be expected.

In practice, the percentage binding of most drugs is less concentration-dependent than Figure 7.3 implies. The concentration scale on the abscissa is logarithmic so that, assuming that n and P are constant, the total concentration range is approximately 10^5, which is far greater than the normal therapeutic range for most drugs. The curves also tend to be horizontal and linear over quite a large proportion of the concentration range, depending on the value of K, so that drug binding to plasma proteins is usually constant and independent of drug concentration, at least within the therapeutic range. Thus, although protein binding should still be taken into account when calculating drug distribution and clearance values, protein binding generally does not affect such parameters as rate constants because they are identical for both the free and total drug.

Disopyramide and phenytoin are exceptions to this rule. The percentage binding of these drugs decreases with increasing drug concentrations in plasma within the therapeutic range (5). For drugs of this type, measurement of free drug concentrations in plasma before attempting to resolve their pharmacokinetics is necessary.

Intravascular and Extravascular Drug Binding

Regardless of the type of plasma protein to which a drug is bound, the effect is always to draw drug into plasma at the expense of other extravascular tissues and fluids. Therefore, if a drug binds to extravascular tissues or proteins, exactly the opposite effect will occur, and drug will be pulled out of plasma. Most drugs that bind to macromolecules to any significant degree are probably affected by both intravascular and extravascular binding. Many different kinds of extravascular molecules are capable of binding drugs, including albumin, fatty tissues, and cell membranes. Extravascular or tissue binding can significantly modulate the effect of drug binding to plasma proteins (6,7).

Earlier in this chapter, drug binding to plasma proteins was considered. The effects of both intravascular and extravascular binding on four major pharmacokinetic parameters will now be examined. These parameters are as follows:

1. The percentage of total drug that is free, or unbound, in the body.

2. The concentration of free drug in plasma.

3. The concentration of total drug in plasma.

4. The apparent distribution volume.

Although in most cases both intravascular and extravascular binding occur simultaneously, they will be considered separately here for convenience and illustration. The concentration of free drug in plasma, C_F, in equilibrium with free drug in other body fluids can be approximated by Equation 7.13.

$$C_F = \frac{A_T}{V_f + 3\gamma + (V_F - 3)\epsilon} \tag{7.13}$$

where A_T is the total amount of drug in the body in milligrams, V_F is the actual distribution volume of free drug in liters; the value 3 is the plasma volume in liters; and γ and ϵ represent the ratios of bound to unbound drug in plasma and in tissue, respectively.

From Equation 7.13, the amount of free drug in the body, A_F, can readily be calculated by Equation 7.14.

$$A_F = C_F V_F \tag{7.14}$$

The concentration of bound drug in plasma, C_B, is obtained from Equation 7.15, the concentration of total drug in plasma, C_T, from Equation 7.16, and the percentage of free drug in the body from Equation 7.17.

$$C_B = C_F \gamma \tag{7.15}$$

$$C_T = C_F + C_B \tag{7.16}$$

$$\text{percent free} = (A_F/A_T) \times 100 \tag{7.17}$$

The apparent distribution volume, V_{app}, is given by Equation 7.18.

$$V_{app} = A_T/C_T \tag{7.18}$$

A simple mathematical example will demonstrate how these equations (7.13–7.18) can be used.

Consider two drugs, A and B. Assume that both drugs distribute into an actual body volume of 20 L, but differ in that at therapeutic concentrations Drug A is 90% bound to plasma proteins and 5% bound to tissue proteins, whereas Drug B is only 5% bound to plasma proteins and 90% bound to tissue proteins. Both drugs are administered so that the total quantity of drug in the body at the time of measurement is 100 mg.

The numerical values for the parameters defined in Equations 7.13–7.18 are calculated in Table 7.6, and the results demonstrate the remarkable effects that binding can have on both real and apparent pharmacokinetic parameters.

For example, the greater overall binding of Drug B, due to the relatively large tissue volume, reduces the concentration of free drug that is in equilibrium and at the same concentration in both plasma and tissue fluids to about one-fourth the concentration of Drug A. The amount of free Drug B in the circulation is also only one-fourth the amount of Drug A, as is the percentage of drug that is free in the body. Although these differences appear large, they are small compared to some other parameters. For example, the concentration of bound drug and, perhaps more importantly for pharmacokinetic calculations, the concentration of total drug in plasma are many times higher for Drug A than for Drug B. The concentration of total Drug A in plasma is 20.9 µg/mL compared to only 0.61 µg/mL for Drug B. Similarly, the apparent distribution volume for Drug A is only 4.8 L (only slightly larger than plasma volume), but the apparent distribution volume of Drug B is 164 L. The true distribution volume for both drugs is 20 L.

These drugs are, of course, two extremes of the possible spectrum of protein-binding combinations, but this example indicates the profound

Table 7.6—Influence of Intravascular and Extravascular Binding on Pharmacokinetic Parameters of Two Drugs, A and B, That Have Different Binding Characteristics

Parameter	Drug A	Drug B
V (actual)	20 L	20 L
A_T	100 mg	100 mg
Percent bound in plasma	90%	5%
Percent bound in tissues ($\mu g/mL$)	5%	90%
C_F ($\mu g/mL$) (Eq. 7.13)	$100/[20 + 3(9) + 17(5/95)] = 2.09$	$100/[20 + 3(5/95) + 17(9)] = 0.58$
A_F (mg) (Eq. 7.14)	$2.09 \times 20 = 41.8$	$0.58 \times 20 = 11.6$
C_B ($\mu g/mL$) (Eq. 7.15)	$2.09 \times 9 = 18.8$	$0.58 \times 5/95 = 0.030$
C_T ($\mu g/mL$) (Eq. 7.16)	$2.09 + 18.8 = 20.9$	$0.58 + 0.030 = 0.61$
Percent free (%) (Eq. 7.17)	$(41.8 \times 100)/100 = 41.8$	$(11.6 \times 100)/100 = 11.6$
V_{app} (L) (Eq. 7.18)	$100/20.9 = 4.8$	$100/0.61 = 163.9$

effect that binding can have on drug distribution, observed plasma levels, and pharmacokinetic parameters.

Consider the percentage of free drug in the body, and how it is affected by plasma and tissue binding. Figure 7.4 describes three hypothetical drugs that have actual distribution volumes of 12, 20, and 42 L. Consider first the effect of variable drug binding to plasma proteins. When plasma binding is zero, the drug is 100% free in the body. When plasma binding is 100%, the drug is 100% bound. However, between these limits the change in the percentage of free drug is not linearly related to protein binding but is curved, and the most rapid changes occur when protein binding exceeds 80–85%. Consider the dashed lines representing tissue binding. As might be expected, the two extremes for these curves are identical to those from the solid lines. Thus, when all the drug is bound, whether in plasma or tissue, no free drug is present in the body. However, in the case of tissue binding, because of the relatively large volume of tissue fluids compared to plasma, (the volume ratio varies from 4:1 to 14:1 for the three drugs considered here), the relationship between the percentage of drug free and bound is almost linear throughout the entire tissue-binding range, and this relationship essentially becomes linear for the drug that has the largest distribution volume of 42 L.

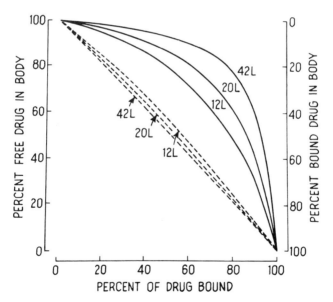

Figure 7.4. Changes in the percentage of drug that is free (unbound) in the body vs. changes in the percentage of circulating drug bound to serum proteins (—) and the percentage of extravascular drug bound to tissues (---). When considering binding at one site (serum protein or tissue), the binding at the other site is assumed to be 0. Curves were generated from Equations 7.13–7.15, $A_T = 100$ mg. The volumes 12, 20, and 42 L represent true distribution volumes of free drug. (Reproduced with permission from reference 6. Copyright 1977, ADIS Australia.)

In Figure 7.5, when binding to plasma proteins is zero, the concentration of free drug (which in this instance will equal the concentration of total drug) in plasma is obtained by dividing the total body load of 100 mg by the actual distribution volume to yield concentrations of 8.3, 5, and 2.4 μg/mL for the drugs with 12-, 20-, and 42-L volumes, respectively. On the other hand, when binding to plasma proteins is 100%, the concentration of free drug is zero; no free drug is present in the body. Between these extremes the concentration of free drug changes only slowly until plasma-protein binding again reaches 80–85%, at which point the concentration drops sharply toward zero as protein binding approaches 100%.

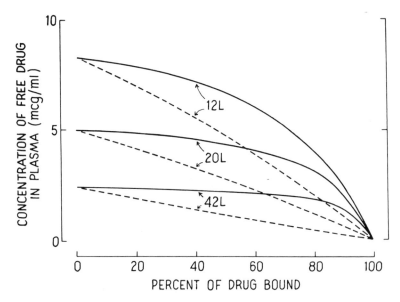

Figure 7.5. Changes in concentration of free drug C_F vs. changes in the percentage of circulating drug bound to plasma proteins (—), and the percentage of extravascular drug bound to tissue (---). Curves were generated from Equation 7.13. Conditions as in Figure 7.4. (Reproduced with permission from reference 6. Copyright 1977, ADIS Australia.)

Tissue binding has the same effect in Figure 7.5 as in Figure 7.4: a virtually linear relationship exists between the free drug concentration and tissue binding, and identical values are obtained when binding to tissue is zero and 100% compared to those values obtained when plasma binding is zero and 100%.

In Figure 7.6, the concentration of total (free and bound) drug in plasma is examined under the same conditions. However, the curves are quite different from the previous figures. At zero binding to plasma protein (left side of the figure), the concentration of total drug in plasma is the same as the concentration of free drug in Figure 7.5. This similarity is reasonable because in both cases there is no bound drug. However, as the degree of binding to plasma proteins increases, the concentration of total drug in plasma also increases until the three solid lines converge to a value of 33.3 µg/mL. This concentration results from all three drugs being totally confined to plasma volume, and the concentration value is determined simply by dividing the total drug load of 100 mg by 3 L. Therefore, although the concentration of free drug decreases with increased plasma-protein binding, the concentration of total drug increases. The changes in total drug concentration (note the alteration in the ordinate values at 10 µg/mL in this figure) increase dramatically after binding exceeds 80%.

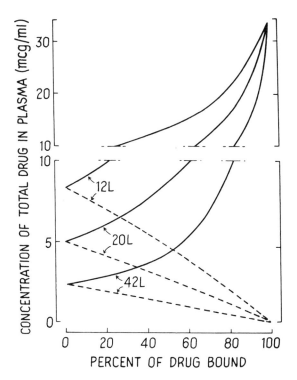

Figure 7.6. Changes in the concentration of total (free and bound) drug in plasma C_T vs. changes in the percentage of circulating drug bound to plasma proteins (—), and the percentage of extravascular drug bound to tissues (- - -). Curves were generated from Equations 7.13–7.18. Conditions were the same as in Figure 4. (Reproduced with permission from reference 6, Copyright 1977, ADIS Australia.)

Tissue binding, on the other hand, has a similar effect on the concentration of total drug to that of free drug. A linear decline in total drug in plasma occurs as drug is bound more extensively to tissues and is drawn out of plasma.

Figure 7.7 describes binding-related changes in the drug apparent distribution volume. The apparent distribution volume value is cited often in the literature but is poorly understood. In this figure, the situation differs dramatically compared to the previous figures.

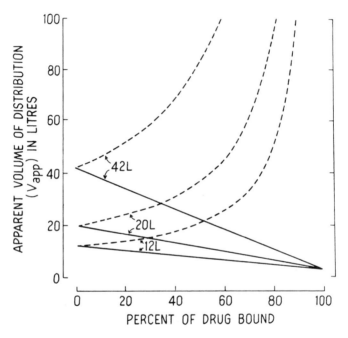

Figure 7.7. Changes in the apparent distribution volume of drug, V_{app}, vs. changes in the percentage of circulating drug bound to plasma proteins (—), and the percentage of extravascular drug bound to tissues (---). Curves were generated from Equations 7.13–7.18. Conditions were the same as in Figure 7.4. (Reproduced with permission from reference 6. Copyright 1977, ADIS Australia.)

The apparent volumes calculated in Figure 7.7 are obtained from Equation 7.18. Apparent volumes are the types of volumes that are generally calculated from total drug levels in plasma. At zero plasma-protein binding (and also at zero tissue binding), the apparent volumes are identical to the true volumes because all of the drug is free. However, as plasma-protein binding increases, the apparent volume decreases linearly to reach a value of 3 L when all of the drug is bound. So, for any degree of drug binding to plasma proteins, the apparent volume of distribution will always underestimate the true volume, and the degree of underestimation will increase as the extent of plasma-protein binding increases.

Tissue binding in this case has the opposite effect on the apparent distribution volume. As the drug binds more avidly to tissues (follow the dashed lines going from left to right in Figure 7.7), the drug is drawn out of the plasma and the drug apparent distribution volume increases to very large values as the concentration of total drug in plasma is reduced. This situation is typical for many drugs. For example, digoxin has an apparent distribution volume seven times greater than body volume, and trimethoprim has an apparent distribution volume approximately double that of body volume. These large apparent volumes of distribution are due to binding or sequestration by tissue that leads to heterogeneous tissue distribution at the expense of plasma levels, and occurs regardless of drug binding to plasma protein. The large apparent distribution volume of trimethoprim relative to that of sulfamethoxazole is the reason that these two drugs are administered in a combination ratio of 5:1 sulfamethoxazole to trimethoprim to achieve a plasma ratio of 20:1 sulfamethoxazole to trimethoprim, which is the optimum ratio for therapeutic effect.

A popular misconception is that if a drug binds to plasma proteins, then the drug cannot penetrate tissues and a small distribution volume results. Certainly, if plasma binding is high and tissue binding is low or zero, then the drug will tend to accumulate in plasma. However, if a drug has affinity for macromolecules, then the drug will tend to bind both in plasma and tissues. Thus, the binding of drugs to plasma and tissue proteins should be related, and a significant correlation between the apparent distribution volume and plasma-protein binding might be expected. Such a correlation has been demonstrated with the four cephalosporin drugs shown in Figure 7.8. Therefore, just because a drug is highly bound to plasma proteins does not mean that the drug cannot penetrate into tissues. Erythromycin is 90% bound to plasma proteins, but only 1–3% of the total body load of this antibiotic is contained within the plasma volume. The remainder of the drug is in tissue.

Figures 7.5 and 7.6 show that changes in the degree of protein binding significantly affect circulating levels of free and total drug only in the binding range of 80% or greater. Many drugs and endogenous substances are capable of displacing other drugs from plasma binding sites and thus alter the unbound–bound equilibrium. However, for all drugs except highly bound molecules, these changes in the unbound–bound equilibrium are likely to be of little pharmacokinetic and clinical significance. Even with highly bound drugs, increases in free drug concentration due to displacement are likely to be rapidly compensated by tissue distribution and elimination of the free drug. Thus, changes in drug concentrations

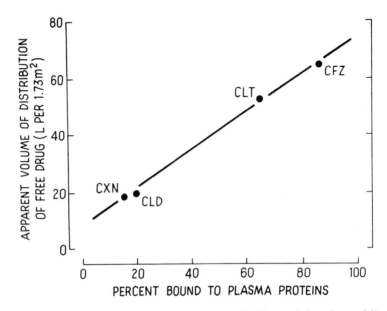

Figure 7.8. Relationship between plasma protein binding and the volume of distribution of free drug for four cephalosporins: CFZ, cefazolin; CLT, cephalothin; CLD, cephaloridine; and CXN, cephalexin. Correlation coefficient = +0.998. (Reproduced with permission from reference 6. Copyright 1977, ADIS Australia.)

due to altered binding are, for the most part, of little clinical significance whether the drug is highly bound or not.

Penetration of Drug into the Central Nervous System (CNS)

The central nervous system (CNS) comprises approximately 2% of body weight, but CNS circulation receives 16% of the cardiac output. Blood flow varies to different regions of the brain. For example, flow to the cortex is 1–2 mL/min per gram, whereas blood flow to cerebral white matter is only 0.24 mL/min per gram.

Surrounding the entire CNS is cerebrospinal fluid (CSF). The CSF has a total volume of about 120 mL, and has a turnover rate of 10–25% per hour. The pathways of CSF flow are shown in Figure 7.9 (8). CSF is formed mainly at the ventricles and choroid plexus in the brain stem, and reenters the general circulation mainly at the arachnoid villi. CSF has a much lower protein content than plasma. CSF serves many purposes, and some of these are as follows:

1. Acting as a hydraulic cushion against brain injury.

2. Maintaining control over ion concentrations in the CNS.

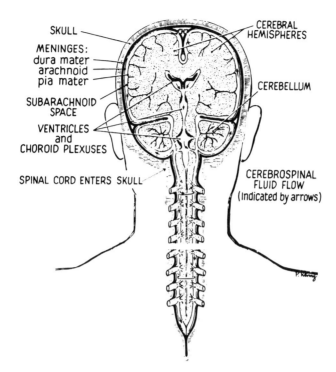

SKULL

MENINGES:
dura mater
arachnoid
pia mater

SUBARACHNOID
SPACE

VENTRICLES
and
CHOROID PLEXUSES

SPINAL CORD ENTERS SKULL

CEREBRAL
HEMISPHERES

CEREBELLUM

CEREBROSPINAL
FLUID FLOW
(Indicated by arrows)

Figure 7.9. Pathways of CSF flow. The flow of CSF from the ventricles to the cerebral and spinal subarachnoid space. (Adapted with permission from reference 8. Copyright 1971, Williams and Wilkins Company.)

   3. Maintaining the CNS at a slightly acidic pH of about 7.2 relative to blood pH of 7.4.

To help in understanding how drugs enter the CNS, Figure 7.10 describes the physical anatomical relationships between blood, CSF, and CNS tissue (8). Drugs can enter the CNS by two different routes, and each route contains a barrier to drug entry. The consequence of these barriers is that, although fat-soluble compounds can readily enter the CNS, water-soluble compounds generally cannot.

   Drugs enter the brain mainly by the indirect route via the CSF. They enter the CSF at the epithelium of the choroid plexus. To enter the CSF from blood, a drug has to pass through the capillary endothelial cells, basement membranes, and stroma. These barriers do not appear to hinder the drug. However, drugs then have to pass through the choroid epithelial cells that appear to contain some type of tight junction that prevents intercellular transport and thus inhibits passage of water-soluble substances. Once within the CSF, no particular barrier is present for drugs to enter the cells of the CNS.

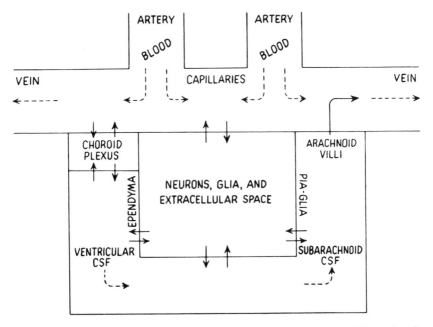

Figure 7.10. Routes by which compounds can enter and leave the CNS (Reproduced with permission from reference 8. Copyright 1971, Williams and Wilkins Company.)

The second route of drug entry into the CNS is directly from the capillaries that constitute the CNS blood supply. In this case, no defense region of the CSF as described for the first route exists. The cells of the capillaries therefore are adapted to provide an alternative and similar defense in the form of glial connective tissue cells (or astrocytes) associated with the basement membrane of the capillary endothelium. Glial connective tissue cells serve a similar purpose to the choroid epithelial cells in restricting entry into the CNS to fat-soluble substances.

Thus two routes for drug entry into the CNS exist, but each route incorporates a defense structure to prevent, or at least minimize, penetration of water-soluble substances. These defense structures constitute the blood–brain barrier.

Drugs generally exit from the CNS either directly into the capillaries or, perhaps more commonly, at the arachnoid villi along with CSF that is reentering the general circulation. Evidence indicates that some compounds, including weak acids and bases, can be removed from CSF by an active process at the choroid plexus.

The efficiency with which the blood–brain barrier works, and the presence of diffusion-limited entry into the CNS, is demonstrated in the classic studies of Brody et al. (9). Some results obtained in these studies are shown in Figure 7.11. The ionization constants, partition coefficients, other physical characteristics, and the entry rate of some drugs into the CSF are listed in Table 7.7 (10). Comparison of these data to Figure 7.11 shows that the rate at which drugs enter the CSF is a function of ionization and lipid–water partitioning. For example, un-ionized salicylic acid (partition coefficient 0.12) partitions into *n*-heptane from water to a greater extent than pentobarbital (partition coefficient 0.05). However, pentobarbital is less ionized at pH 7.4. Therefore, pentobarbital has an effective partition coefficient, and hence diffusion rate into the CSF from plasma, greater than that of salicylic acid.

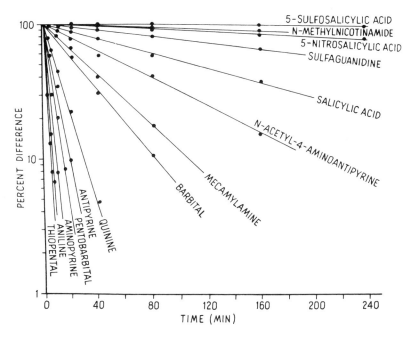

Figure 7.11. Rate of equilibration of various drugs between plasma and CSF. (Figure reproduced with permission from reference 10. Copyright 1980, Lea and Febiger. Data from reference 9.)

Many antibiotics are water-soluble and do not enter the brain very efficiently. However, in some infections such as meningitis, the permeability of the CNS and CSF membranes increases, allowing more compounds to enter the CNS. This phenomenon has been noted for such drugs as ampicillin, penicillin G, cephalosporins, and lincomycin. Increased drug penetration into the CNS has also been noted in some experimental studies concerning brain tumors. The development of compounds, prodrugs, and drug delivery techniques that will penetrate the blood–brain barrier and provide therapeutic drug levels in the brain con-

Table 7.7—Properties of Drugs and Times to Reach 50% Equilibrium Concentration Values Between Plasma and CSF

Drug	Fraction Bound to Protein at pH 7.4	pK$_a$	Fraction Un-ionized at pH 7.4	Partition Coefficient (n-Heptane–Water) of Un-ionized Form	Effective Partition Coefficient	Time to Reach 50% Equilibrium Between Plasma and CSF (min)
Thiopental	0.75	7.6	0.61	3.3	2.0	1.4
Aminopyrine	0.20	5.0	1.0	0.21	0.21	2.8
Pentobarbital	0.40	8.1	0.83	0.05	0.042	4.0
Antipyrine	0.08	1.4	1.0	0.005	0.005	5.8
Barbital	<0.02	7.5	0.56	0.002	0.001	27.0
N-Acetyl-4-aminoantipyrine	<0.03	0.5	1.0	0.001	0.001	56.0
Salicylic acid	0.4	3.0	0.004	0.12	0.0005	115.0
Sulfaguanidine	0.06	>10.0	1.0	<0.001	<0.001	231.0

SOURCE: Adapted from reference 10.

tinues to challenge the ingenuity of pharmaceutical chemists and formulators.

Summary

1. Capillary membranes are more permeable than most other physiological membranes to most compounds. Lipophilic molecules tend to cross the membranes readily. The ease with which hydrophilic compounds cross capillary membranes is inversely proportional to the molecular weight of the compounds.

2. Drug distribution into tissues may be perfusion or diffusion rate limited.

3. Drug binding to plasma proteins can be characterized mathematically in terms of drug concentration, affinity, and the number of binding sites on the protein molecule.

4. The free drug concentration in the body, the concentration of free drug in serum (or plasma), and the concentration of total drug in serum are related in a nonlinear fashion to plasma-protein binding.

5. Changes in plasma-protein binding have a significant effect on drug distribution and drug levels in plasma only when the drug is highly bound, or when changes occur in the highly bound state.

6. The apparent distribution volume of a drug is markedly dependent on plasma-protein and tissue binding. Plasma-protein binding tends

to reduce the apparent volume, and tissue binding tends to increase the apparent volume relative to the true volume.

7. Both the degree of ionization and the lipid–water partition coefficient are important determinants of drug entry into the CNS. For many drugs, passage from blood to brain is diffusion rate limited. Low permeability of membranes separating the circulation from the CSF or CNS to water-soluble compounds represents the blood–brain barrier.

Literature Cited

1. Creasey, W. A. *Drug Disposition in Humans: The Basis of Clinical Pharmacology;* Oxford University: New York, 1979, pp 33–54.
2. Smith, C. G.; Reineke, L. M.; Burch, M. R.; Shefner, A. M.; Muirhead, E. E. *Cancer Research,* **1970,** *30,* 69–75.
3. Goldstein, A.; Aranow, L.; Kalman, S. M. *Principles of Drug Action: The Basis of Pharmacology,* 2nd ed.; John Wiley: New York, 1974, pp 130–138.
4. Rowland, M.; Tozer, T. N. *Clinical Pharmacokinetics: Concepts and Applications;* Lea and Febiger: Philadelphia, 1980.
5. Meffin, P. J.; Robert, E. W.; Winkle, R. A.; Harapat, S.; Peters, F. A.; Harrison, D. C. *J. Pharmacokin. Biopharm.* **1979,** *7,* 29–42.
6. Craig, W. A.; Welling, P. G. *Clin. Pharmacokin.* **1977,** *2,* 252–268.
7. Craig, W. A.; Kunin, C. M. *Annu. Rev. Med.* **1976,** *27,* 287–300.
8. Rall, D. In *Fundamentals of Drug Metabolism and Drug Disposition;* La Du, B. N.; Mandel, H. G.; Way, El. L.; Eds.; Williams and Wilkins: Baltimore, 1981, pp 76–87.
9. Brodie, B. B.; Kurtz, H.; Schanker, L. S. *J. Pharmacol. Exp. Therap.* **1960,** *130,* 20–25.
10. Rowland, M.; Tozer, T. N. *Clinical Pharmacokinetics, Concepts and Applications;* Lea and Febiger: Philadelphia; 1980, pp 34–47.

Problems

1. A dose of 250 mg of a drug is administered to a 70-kg male patient by rapid intravenous injection. The concentration of total drug in plasma 5 min after injection is 20.8 $\mu g/mL$. Calculate the apparent distribution volume of the drug assuming that the drug does not bind to plasma proteins and loss of drug from the body during the first 5 min is negligible.

2. Recalculate the distribution volume from the previous question assuming that:
(i) The drug is 70% bound to plasma proteins, and also that
(ii) The drug is eliminated at such a rate that 20% of the dose is excreted from the body during the initial 5 min after dosing.

3. A drug has a true distribution volume in the body of 42 L. The drug is 90% bound to plasma proteins and 0% bound in tissue. Calculate the values of C_F, C_B, C_T, A_F, and V_{app} for the drug when the total body load is 100 mg.

4. Recalculate the values in Problem 3 on the basis that the drug is 90% bound to plasma proteins and 80% bound in tissue.

5. Recalculate the values in Problem 3 on the basis that plasma-protein binding is reduced to 60% and tissue binding remains unchanged at 80%.

8

Drug Metabolism

The metabolism of drugs and other foreign substances can be considered part of the body's natural defense mechanisms that defend the homeostatic balance of the system against the invasion of foreign substances.

Although drug metabolism has been recognized for some considerable time, the study of drug metabolism first became an organized and well-defined scientific endeavor through the pioneering work and dedication of the late R. Tecwyn Williams. His book, *Detoxication Mechanisms*, published in 1959, still serves as an authoritative text on the routes of metabolism of drugs and other chemicals (1). The title indicates one of the major natural functions of drug metabolism, which is the formation of more water-soluble derivatives of parent compounds. This derivatization usually results in loss of pharmacological activity and more rapid excretion. Bernard B. Brodie once said, "If there were no such process as drug metabolism, it would take the body about 100 years to terminate the action of pentobarbital, which is lipid-soluble and cannot be excreted without being metabolized."

All of the reactions involved in drug metabolism are adaptations of biochemical, enzymatic processes that were in existence long before drugs were synthesized. The enzymes that oxidize phenobarbital or demethylate codeine, for example, were in existence in the body long before these drugs were discovered. The biochemical systems have adapted to cope with these new compounds, but were not created for these purposes.

0065-7719/86/0185-0103$06.00/1
© 1986 American Chemical Society

Sites of Drug Metabolism

Drug metabolism takes place in many parts of the body. Metabolism can occur in the bloodstream, spleen, kidneys, brain, muscle tissue, the contents (bacteria) and wall of the GI tract, and many other tissues. The prostaglandins, for example, are extensively metabolized in lung tissue. However, the major organ in which drug metabolism takes place is the liver. The liver is the primary organ of waste disposal and works in close collaboration with the kidneys to eliminate unwanted substances from the body.

The liver is the largest gland in the body and weighs 1.2–1.6 kg. The liver receives blood from the region of the GI tract, spleen, and gall bladder via the portal vein; it receives blood from the aorta via the hepatic artery. Approximately 80% of the total hepatic blood flow of 1.5 L/min is supplied by the portal vein. After entering the liver, the portal vein divides into a rich capillary network of hepatic sinusoids. Kupffer cells are found in the walls of the sinusoids. Blood penetrates into the liver parenchymal cells from the sinusoids through fine intracellular caniculi.

The sinusoids converge toward the center of the liver lobule to form sublobular veins. Sublobular veins combine to form hepatic veins that rejoin the general circulation at the inferior vena cava. This unique hepatic vascular architecture provides intimate contact between substances being transported in portal blood and the hepatic parenchymal cells.

Around each portal vein branch is a plexus of bile capillaries. Bile capillaries enter into interlobular bile ducts that eventually combine to form the hepatic duct. In humans and higher mammals, bile is stored in the gall bladder before entering the duodenum via the common bile duct.

The hepatic artery is primarily responsible for oxygenation of the liver. Although this artery supplies only 20% of total hepatic blood flow, the greater part of the oxygen supplied to the liver is provided by the hepatic artery.

The site within the liver parenchymal cell where most metabolism takes place is the microsomal fraction, or *microsomes*. Microsomes is a name given to a liver fraction obtained by sequential centrifugation of homogenized liver. More specifically, liver is homogenized at 9000 g, the precipitate discarded, and the supernate centrifuged at 100,000 g. The resulting precipitate is the microsomal fraction.

The microsomal fraction is derived from the endoplasmic reticulum, which is a subcellular component. The two types of endoplasmic reticulum are designated according to their microscopic appearance and activity: rough-surfaced or smooth-surfaced. The rough-surfaced form contains the ribosomes and ribonucleoproteins that are involved in protein synthesis. The drug-metabolizing enzymes are associated primarily with the smooth-surfaced endoplasmic reticulum, although other sites of metabolism are known. For example, alcohol dehydrogenase is located primarily in the soluble fraction of the hepatocyte.

Alteration of drugs by the biochemical processes of the body tends to reduce pharmacological activity and increase the elimination rate of drugs. The loss of pharmacological activity is relatively simple to understand because the metabolite in most cases is not only more water-soluble than the parent drug, and therefore less capable of crossing membranes (for example, the blood–brain barrier), but the metabolite has also lost most of the original intrinsic pharmacological activity. Medicinal chemists know only too well that pharmacological activity is very specific for molecular structure.

The most important consequence of drug metabolism is the increased aqueous solubility of metabolites compared to the parent drug. As will be described (Chapter 9), drugs that reach the kidneys in the bloodstream are subject to three major processes: filtration from blood into the kidney tubules at the glomerulus, active secretion from blood into the proximal convoluting tubules of the kidney, and passive reabsorption back into the bloodstream from the distal convoluting tubules. The filtration and active-secretion mechanisms have their own particular characteristics, but these mechanisms are not sensitive to fat solubility, unless fat solubility affects some other parameter. Passive reabsorption, on the other hand, is restricted to lipophilic substances that are capable of crossing the membranes that line the distal tubules and thereby reenter the general circulation.

By converting a drug into a more water-soluble form (a metabolite), drug metabolism prevents distal tubular reabsorption from occurring and thereby promotes renal excretion. Metabolites may also be cleared by other routes including the lungs, bile, saliva, and sweat, but renal elimination is the most important route in most cases.

Although drug metabolism usually produces more water-soluble compounds, in some cases the metabolites are less water-soluble than the parent drug. Good examples of this phenomenon can be found among the sulfonamides. This group of antimicrobial agents has a common basic structure, and sulfonamides are metabolized primarily by acetylation at the free amino group. This acetylation usually produces a more water-soluble derivative, as shown in Table 8.1. The aqueous solubility of the N-acetyl derivatives of sulfathiazole and sulfacetamide is less than that of the parent drugs, but the solubility of sulfapyrazine is unchanged, and that of sulfamerazine is increased. The occurrence of crystalurea is clearly related to the aqueous solubilities of the drugs and their metabolites. Patients taking such drugs are advised to drink plenty of water to flush the kidneys and thereby prevent crystal deposition.

Other interesting examples of decreased aqueous solubility that leads to longer duration of metabolites in the body compared to the parent

Table 8.1—Aqueous Solubility of Some Sulfonamides and Their Acetylated Metabolites Along with Occurrence of Crystal Deposits in Kidney

Drug	Aqueous Solubility of Drug at 37°C (mg%)	Aqueous Solubility of N-Acetyl Derivative at 37°C (mg%)	Occurrence of Crystal Deposits in Kidney
Sulfathiazole	98	7	Very frequent
Sulfapyrazine	5	5	Very frequent
Sulfamerazine	37	79	Frequent
Sulfacetamide	1100	215	None

drug are desmethyldiazepam and desmethylmethsuximide, both of which have longer plasma elimination half-lives than the parent drugs diazepam and methsuximide.

Mechanisms of Drug Metabolism

Drug metabolism reactions occur in two distinct phases, Phase I and Phase II. Some drugs participate in both phases, other drugs undergo either Phase I or Phase II metabolism. Some examples are given in Scheme 8.1.

Phase I Mechanisms. During Phase I, compounds are chemically activated, mainly by oxidation but also by reduction, or hydrolysis. This process could be considered as putting a chemical handle on a compound to prepare it for a possible Phase II reaction. These chemical activation reactions may result in pharmacological activation, for example, chloral hydrate oxidation; change of activity, for example, codeine demethylation to form morphine; or loss of pharmacological activity, for example, hydroxylation of phenobarbital. The last classification, loss of pharmacological activity, is the most common.

Phase II reactions are different from Phase I reactions because Phase II reactions involve chemical conjugation or synthesis. Actually, very few conjugation reactions exist for Phase II reactions, but these reactions act upon an enormous variety of substrates. Phase II reactions also generally increase water solubility, but there are exceptions. At one time, all Phase II reactions were considered to be pharmacologically deactivating, but this hypothesis is now known to be false. For example, procainamide is acetylated by a Phase II mechanism to form N-acetylprocainamide, which has similar pharmacological activity to the parent drug.

For a Phase II conjugation reaction to occur, a compound must be chemically prepared or chemically active. For drugs i through iii in Scheme 8.1, this preparation is achieved in these particular examples by a Phase I reaction that provides free hydroxyl groups. If a compound is already

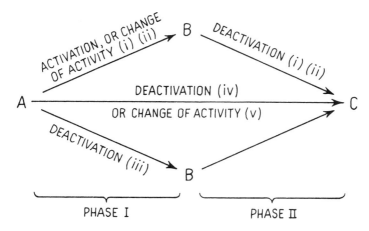

Scheme 8.1. The two major phases of drug metabolism.

Examples:

	A		B		C
i	chloral hydrate	activation ⟶	trichlorethanol	deactivation ⟶	glucuronide
ii	codeine	change of activity ⟶	morphine	deactivation ⟶	glucuronide
iii	phenobarbital	deactivation ⟶	p-OH-phenobarbital	⟶	glucuronide
iv	sulfanilamide	deactivation ⟶			acetate
v	procainamide	change of activity ⟶			acetate

chemically active (chemical activity is not related in any way to pharmacological activity), then the compound may undergo a Phase II reaction directly because the Phase I step is unnecessary. Two examples of compounds that take this route are sulfanilamide and procainamide.

Further examples of the major Phase I oxidation reactions are described in detail in Schemes 8.2–8.9.

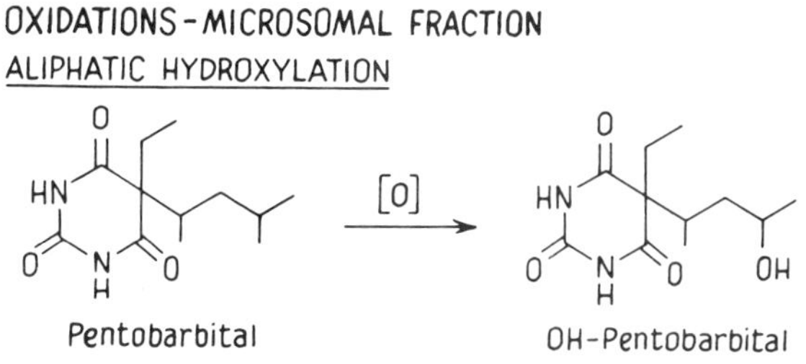

OXIDATIONS – MICROSOMAL FRACTION
ALIPHATIC HYDROXYLATION

Pentobarbital   [O] ⟶   OH-Pentobarbital

Scheme 8.2

AROMATIC HYDROXYLATION

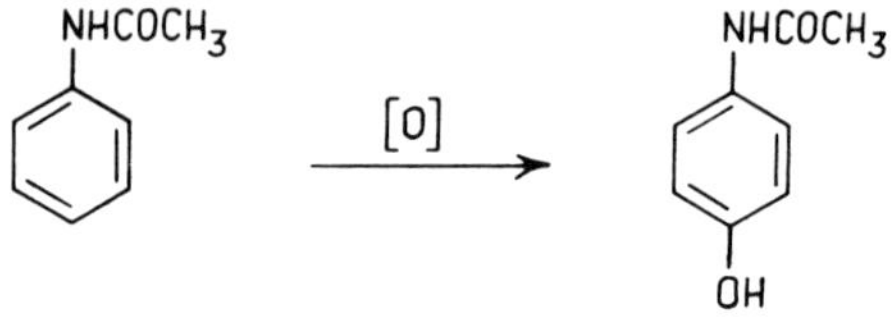

Acetanilide   P-OH-Acetanilide

Scheme 8.3

N-DEALKYLATION

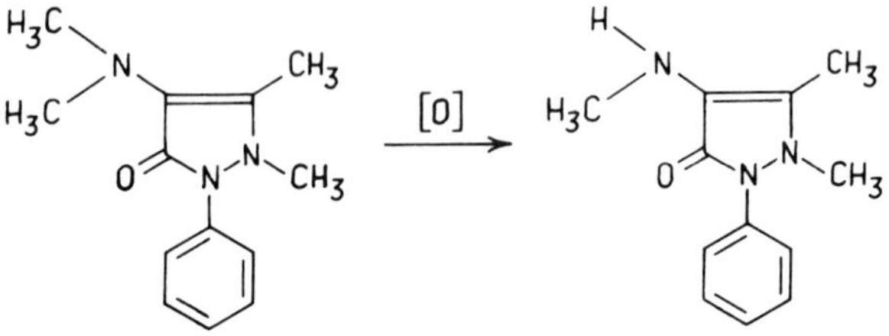

Aminopyrine   Methyl-4-Aminoantipyrine

Scheme 8.4

O-DEALKYLATION

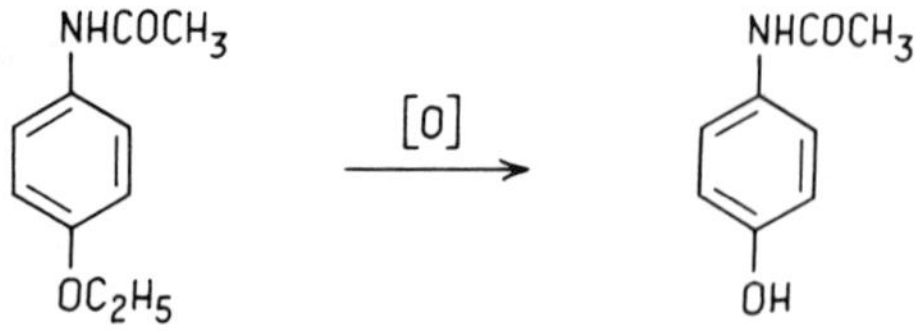

Phenacetin   p-OH-Acetanilide

Scheme 8.5

OXIDATIVE DEAMINATION

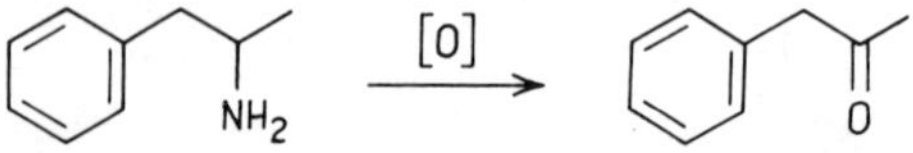

Amphetamine   Phenylacetone

Scheme 8.6

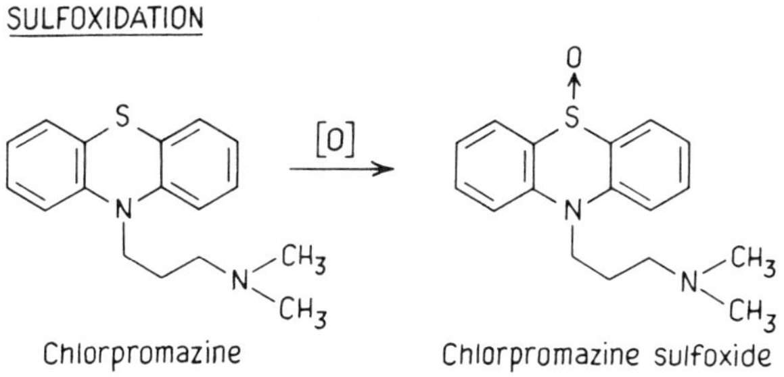

SULFOXIDATION

Chlorpromazine   Chlorpromazine sulfoxide

Scheme 8.7

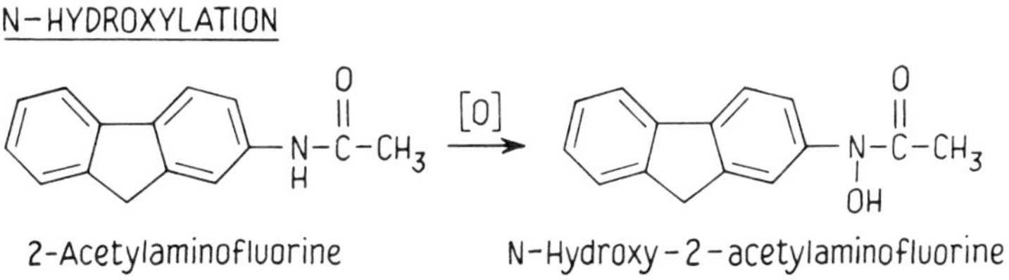

N-HYDROXYLATION

2-Acetylaminofluorine   N-Hydroxy-2-acetylaminofluorine

Scheme 8.8

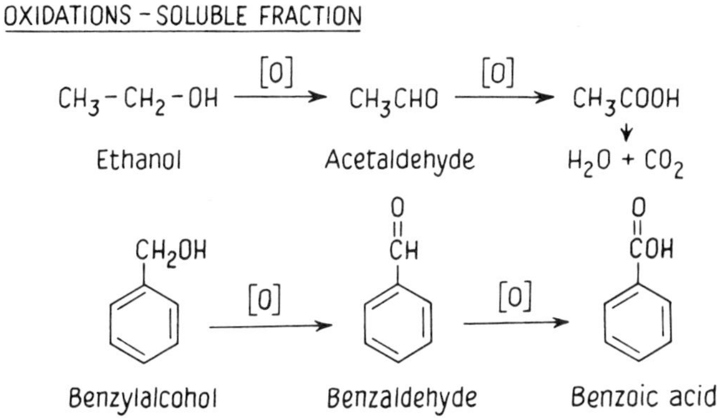

OXIDATIONS - SOLUBLE FRACTION

$$CH_3-CH_2-OH \xrightarrow{[O]} CH_3CHO \xrightarrow{[O]} CH_3COOH$$

Ethanol   Acetaldehyde $\downarrow$
                                          $H_2O + CO_2$

Benzylalcohol   Benzaldehyde   Benzoic acid

Scheme 8.9

The Phase I oxidation reactions include the following: Aliphatic and aromatic hydroxylation, N- and O-dealkylation, Oxidative deamination, Sulfoxidation, and N-hydroxylation.

All of these reactions take place in the microsomal cell fraction, the endoplasmic reticulum. Alcohol dehydrogenase, on the other hand, occurs in the soluble cell fraction. Ethyl alcohol and benzyl alcohol are two typical substrates for this reaction.

The ease with which a drug undergoes oxidative reactions, or any other metabolic reaction, may profoundly influence the biological half-life of the drug in the body. The two hypoglycemic agents, chlorpropamide and tolbutamide, have similar pharmacological activity. These agents also have similar chemical structures, except that tolbutamide has an additional methylene group in the side chain and also a methyl group *para* on the benzene ring, but chlorpropamide has a chloro group *para* on the ring (*see* structures). The methyl group on tolbutamide is readily metabolized sequentially through the alcohol and the aldehyde to the carboxylic acid, which is then conjugated. The chloro group on chlorpropamide, on the other hand, is resistant to metabolism. Thus, tolbutamide has a biological half-life in the body of approximately 4 h compared to 10–12 h for chlorpropamide, and therefore tolbutamide has to be dosed more frequently in clinical practice.

Tolbutamide

$$H_3C-\!\!\!\!\bigcirc\!\!\!\!-\underset{\underset{O}{\downarrow}}{\overset{\overset{O}{\uparrow}}{S}}-\underset{H}{N}-\overset{\overset{O}{\parallel}}{C}-\underset{H}{N}-(CH_2)_3-CH_3$$

Chlorpropamide

$$Cl-\!\!\!\!\bigcirc\!\!\!\!-\underset{\underset{O}{\downarrow}}{\overset{\overset{O}{\uparrow}}{S}}-\underset{H}{N}-\overset{\overset{O}{\parallel}}{C}-\underset{H}{N}-(CH_2)_2-CH_3$$

There are only two major Phase I reduction reactions, nitro reduction and azo reduction, as shown in Schemes 8.10 and 8.11. Mammalian livers carry out these reactions far less effectively than the intestinal microflora. Therefore, Phase I reduction reactions tend to occur more commonly when drugs are administered orally.

The last major Phase I mechanism is hydrolysis. Esterases are ubiquitous enzymes that are active in plasma and other tissues as well as the liver. Esterases are capable of hydrolyzing a large number of esters to alcohols and free carboxylic acids. The example in Scheme 8.12 is interesting because the rapid in vivo hydrolysis of procaine, a compound originally used for cardiac arrhythmias, led to the development of procainamide. The amide is more resistant to hydrolysis than the ester, and is therefore a far more useful drug. As already noted, procainamide is metabolized predominantly by acetylation rather than by hydrolysis.

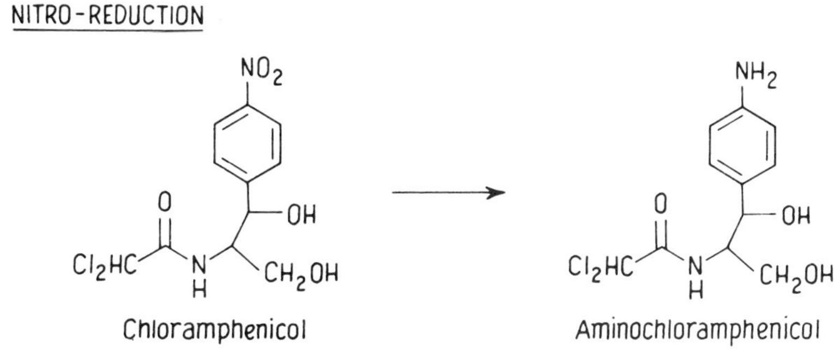
NITRO-REDUCTION
NO_2
O
OH
Cl_2HC
N
H
CH_2OH
Chloramphenicol
NH_2
O
OH
Cl_2HC
N
H
CH_2OH
Aminochloramphenicol

Scheme 8.10

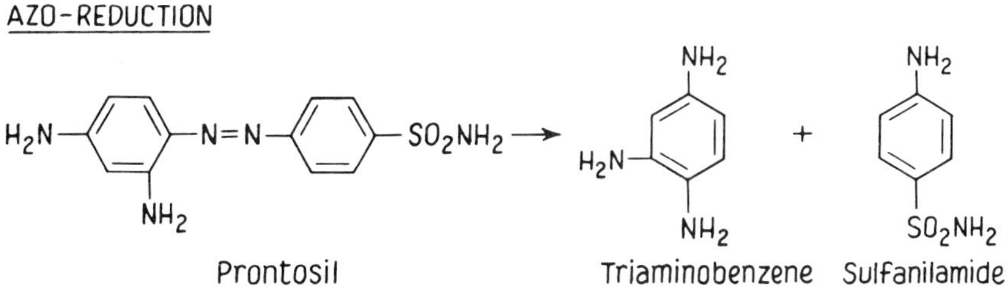
AZO-REDUCTION
H_2N
N=N
SO_2NH_2
NH_2
Prontosil
NH_2
H_2N
NH_2
Triaminobenzene
+
NH_2
SO_2NH_2
Sulfanilamide

Scheme 8.11

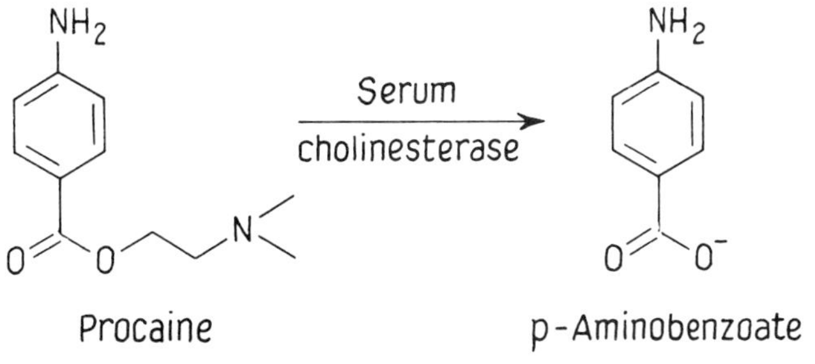
NH_2
O
O
N
Procaine
Serum
cholinesterase
NH_2
O
O^-
p-Aminobenzoate

Scheme 8.12

Mechanism of Oxidative Drug Metabolism. A key element in the oxidative process is the hemoprotein, cytochrome P–450. This was so named for the development of an absorption peak at 450 nm when the hemoprotein reacts with carbon monoxide. Cytochrome P–450 plays a vital role in an electron-transport system in which electrons are lost by the drug during oxidation and passed along an electron-transport system to the final receptor NADPH (nicotine adenosine dinucleotide phosphate). In this process, "active oxygen," which is instrumental in the oxidative process, is generated. The role of cytochrome P–450 in oxidative metabolism, as currently understood, is shown in Scheme 8.13. NADPH acts conversely as an electron donor in a reverse process for reductive metabolic reactions (2,3).

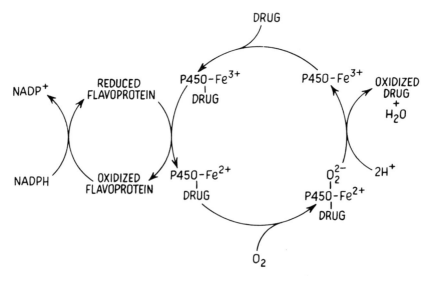

Scheme 8.13. Outline of the electron transport chain involving cytochrome P–450 and the oxidation of drugs by the hepatic microsomal system. Adapted from references 2 and 3.

Phase II Mechanisms. Examples of Phase II conjugation reactions are given in Schemes 8.14–8.19. Unlike Phase I reactions, where a large variety of different reactions may occur, Phase II reactions are relatively few, the principal ones leading to formation of the following compounds:

- Glucuronides of phenols, alcohols, carboxylic acids, and aromatic amines.
- Acetates of amines and sulfonamides.
- Sulfates, mainly of phenols.

- Glycine conjugates of aromatic carboxylic acids.

- Mercapturic acid conjugates of aromatic hydrocarbons, halogenated hydrocarbons, and halogenated nitrobenzenes.

- N-, S-, and O-methylation of phenols, amines, and sulfhydryl compounds.

GLUCURONIDES

Occurs with phenols, alcohols, carboxylic acids, aromatic amines

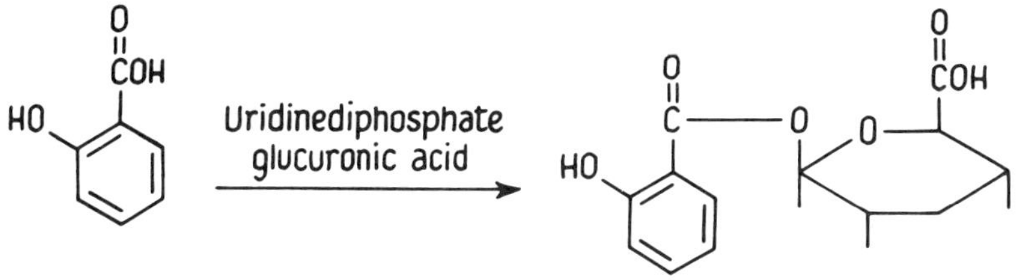

Salicylic acid   Salicylic acid glucuronide

Scheme 8.14

ACYLATION

Occurs with amines, sulfonamides

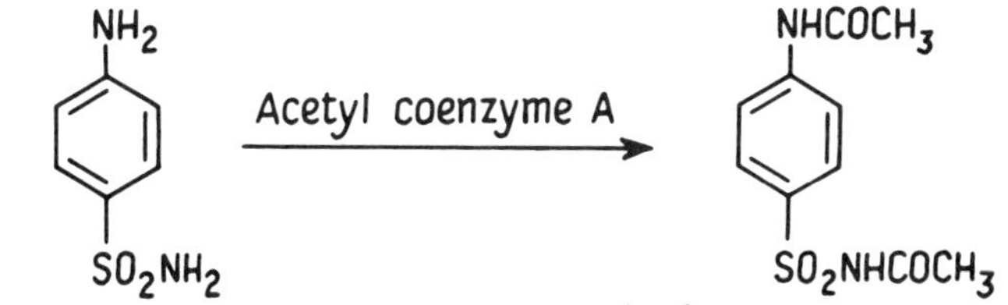

Sulfanilamide N^1, N^4-diacetylsulfanilamide

Scheme 8.15

SULFATION

Occurs mainly with phenols

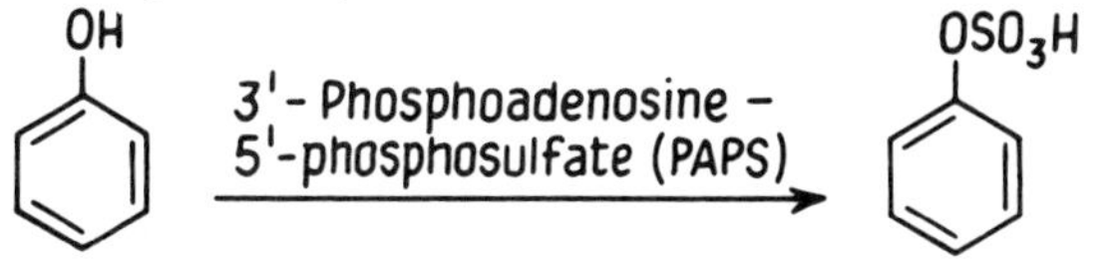

Phenol   Phenyl sulfate

Scheme 8.16

GLYCINE CONJUGATION

Occurs with aromatic carboxylic acids

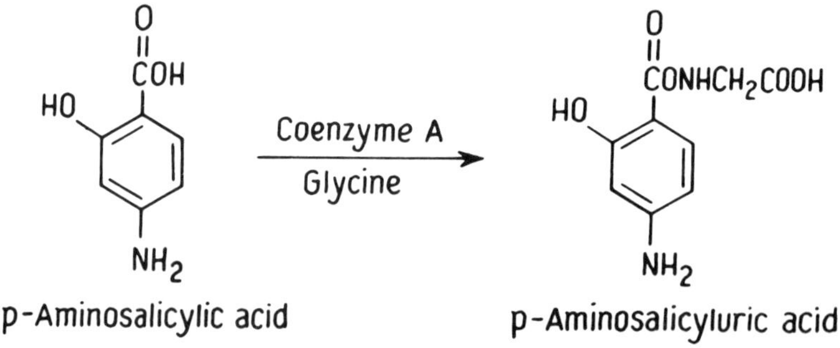
O
COH
HO
NH_2
Coenzyme A
Glycine
O
$CONHCH_2COOH$
HO
NH_2
p-Aminosalicylic acid
p-Aminosalicyluric acid

Scheme 8.17

MERCAPTURIC ACIDS

Occurs with aromatic hydrocarbons, halogenated hydrocarbons, and halogenated aromatic hydrocarbons

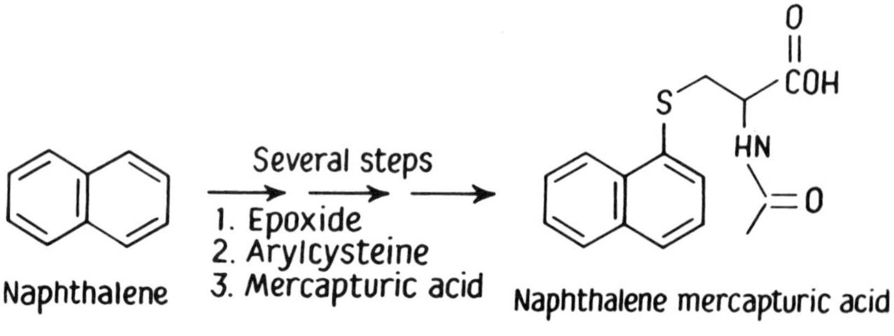
Several steps
1. Epoxide
2. Arylcysteine
3. Mercapturic acid
O
COH
S
HN
O
Naphthalene
Naphthalene mercapturic acid

Scheme 8.18

The conjugation steps, which are each specific for particular functional groups and under the control of a specific enzyme system, represent the final stage in the preparation of compounds for removal from the body. Phase II reactions generally reduce or completely inhibit pharmacological activity and also increase aqueous solubility. The acetylation of procainamide is one of the exceptions to this rule. Thus, Phase II reactions collectively represent a sophisticated and efficient process for terminating the activity of many drugs and removing them from the body. The formation of glycine conjugates tends to be more saturable than most other conjugation reactions because the formation depends on the availability of free glycine in the body.

These mechanisms represent the most common drug metabolism reactions. Other systems may be specific for particular compounds, for example, the action of xanthine oxidase in purine metabolism, and also the formation of nucleotides of some antineoplastic agents. Detailed discussion of these reactions is beyond the scope of this book, but additional material on these subjects is available (4–7).

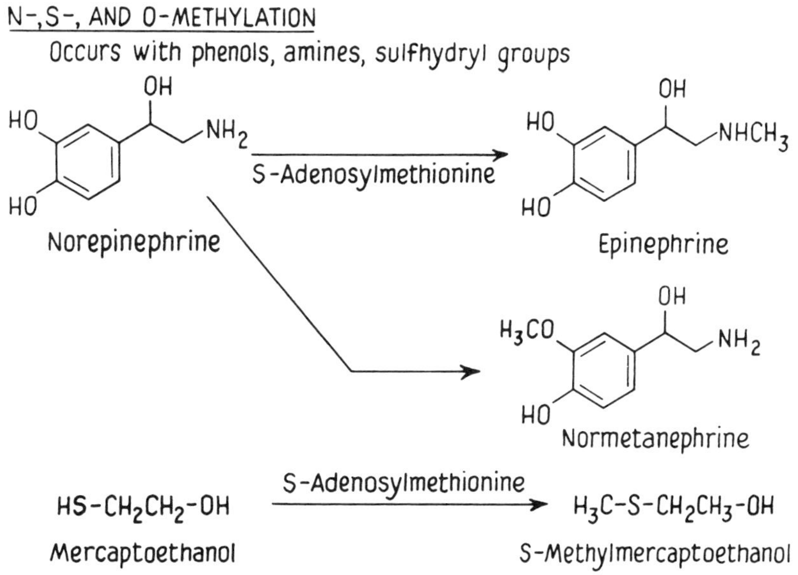

N-,S-, AND O-METHYLATION
Occurs with phenols, amines, sulfhydryl groups

Scheme 8.19

Species, Sex, and Age Differences

When considering drug metabolism, particularly during the development of a new drug, determining how constant the metabolic processes are within and between species is important. Within a species, the reactions are generally qualitatively similar, and only quantitative differences that are expected with normal biological variation are observed. However, some exceptions do occur. For example, a 36-fold range in plasma levels of desmethylimipramine has been reported in patients receiving identical doses of imipramine. Vesell (8) examined the metabolic rates and plasma half-lives of several drugs including antipyrine, bishydroxycoumarin, and phenylbutazone in fraternal and identical twins. The differences between fraternal twins were between 6 and 22 times greater than between pairs of identical twins. This difference represents a good example of genetic, rather than environmental, causes of different metabolic rates. Probably the best example of genetically based variation in drug metabolism is the rate of acetylation of isoniazid and some other compounds. This metabolic step is distinctly bimodal between "fast" and "slow" acetylators. Interestingly, Caucasian and black populations appear to have a predominance of slow acetylators, whereas orientals, Eskimos, and American indians appear to have a predominance of fast acetylators. Tests have been described to identify fast and slow acetylators, and these tests facilitate accurate dosing of isoniazid for the treatment of tuberculosis.

Some sex differences in drug metabolism have been observed in experimental animals, but these differences appear to be negligible in humans. This observation is important in view of the policies of many regulatory agencies that conduct drug absorption and pharmacokinetic studies in male subjects only.

Age can play an important role in the rate of drug metabolism, but only in the very young and very old. A very long plateau exists from early childhood well into old age during which drug metabolism efficiency is fairly constant. In the very young, newborn, and even in the fetus, the lack or immaturity of drug-metabolizing enzymes may constitute a problem. This problem is particularly important for the unborn child because drugs frequently cross the placenta efficiently so that whatever the mother ingests, the fetus will probably receive, too. Typically, the ingestion of alcohol and nicotine has been shown to cause severe effects in the fetus. Other drugs may give rise to adverse effects in the fetus because of impaired metabolism or other mechanisms, and these drugs include some narcotic and nonnarcotic analgesics, benzodiazepines, local anesthetics, neuromuscular blocking agents, anticholinergics, antithyroid drugs, hypoglycemic agents, anticoagulants, and some antimicrobials (9,10).

If species are compared, the picture changes. Profound qualitative and quantitative species differences in metabolism may exist from one species to another. For example, a mitochondrial enzyme system in the guinea pig and the rat converts cyclohexanecarboxylic acid to benzoic acid, whereas this aromatizing activity is absent from most other species, including humans. Another example of species differences affecting drug metabolism is the formation of glutamine conjugates of some acids by humans and apes, but not by other species. Birds and reptiles use ornithine in place of glutamine and glycine for conjugation of carboxylic acids. Dogs cannot acetylate as efficiently as most other species.

Other species differences affecting drug metabolism of a more quantitative nature are abundant. Many drugs have far longer biological half-lives in humans than in other species. For example, the plasma half-life of phenylbutazone is between 2 and 3 days in humans but only 6 h in dogs and guinea pigs, and only 3 h in rabbits. This difference appears to be due to slower reduction of cytochrome P–450 in humans. On the other hand, acetylation of aromatic amines is much faster in humans than in dogs. The primary route of ephedrine metabolism in dogs and guinea pigs is N-demethylation to norephedrine, whereas in rats and humans, norephedrine is only a minor metabolite. Humans metabolize epineph-rine primarily to 3-methoxy-4-hydroxymandelic acid, along with conjugated metanephrine. Cats, on the other hand, convert epinephrine primarily to 3-methoxy-4-hydroxyphenylglycol. Rats form both of these metabolites.

These few examples illustrate the inherent dangers in extrapolating drug metabolism, pharmacokinetics, and toxicity data from experimental animals to humans unless the relative behavior of drug in the different species has been established.

Enzyme Induction

The rate at which an experimental animal or human metabolizes a drug is not always constant. A number of drugs can increase the activity of drug-metabolizing enzymes. These drugs include pentobarbital, phen-obarbital, the carcinogenic hydrocarbon benzo[a]pyrene, steroid hor-mones, ethyl alcohol, the anticonvulsant carbamazepine, and nicotine. These drugs may also stimulate their own metabolism; this process is called *autoinduction*. For example, chronic dosing of the anticonvulsant methsuximide can lead to induction of oxidative demethylation to the active metabolite desmethylmethsuximide.

If a drug is cleared from the body in unchanged form, prior exposure to the drug or to enzyme inducers is unimportant. However, for a drug that is metabolized, it is important to avoid, or at least be cognizant of, the possibility of prior drug exposure when establishing baseline meta-bolic or pharmacokinetic patterns, or dose–response relationships.

Enzyme induction occurs primarily after repeated administration of the inducing agent and is associated with increased liver weight and protein content. Liver concentrations of cytochrome P–450, NADPH–cytochrome C reductase, and cytochrome b_5 also increase. Present evidence suggests that induction involves changes in the enzymes that are part of the drug-metabolizing microsomal system, rather than changes in the rate of NADPH generation.

Enzyme Inhibition

Drug-metabolizing enzymes can also be inhibited, and these effects tend to be more acute and more immediate than induction. Inhibition appears to be the result of direct competition between compounds for drug metabolizing enzymes. The compound β-diethylaminoethyl diphenylpro-pylacetate (SKF 525A, Structure I) is a potent enzyme inhibitor. Compound I has little pharmacological effect of its own, but has the remarkable property of competitively inhibiting the metabolism of a large number of drugs, thereby increasing their biological half-lives and duration of pharmacological effect of these other drugs. The inhibitory effect of Compound I is not limited to oxidation because azo reduction and nitro reduction, which require NADPH but not active oxygen, are also inhibited by this compound. Compound I is thus a powerful pharmacological tool for the study of drug metabolism, but it is not used clinically. Other compounds that inhibit drug-metabolizing enzymes include allopurinol, chloramphenicol, warfarin, and monoamine oxidase inhibitors.

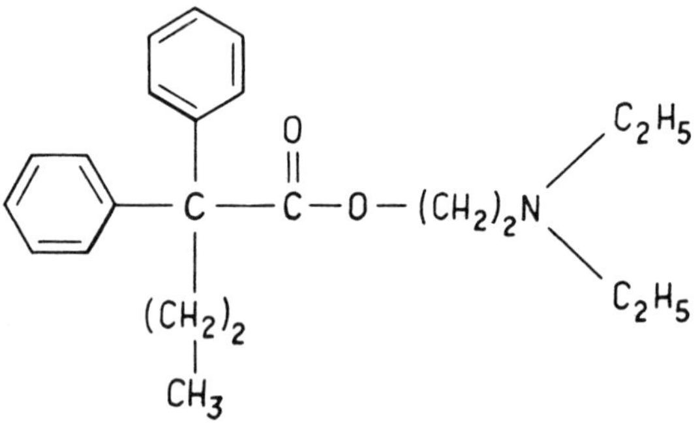

Structure I

An interesting example of the use of drug inhibition in clinical practice is that of disulfiram for the treatment of alcoholism. This compound (Structure II) also has no useful pharmacological activity alone but is capable of blocking alcohol oxidation at the aldehyde step. This blocking causes accumulation of acetylaldehyde in the body after ethyl alcohol ingestion that leads to a violently unpleasant syndrome that includes nausea and vomiting. Disulfiram is used under medical supervision to deter alcohol consumption by association.

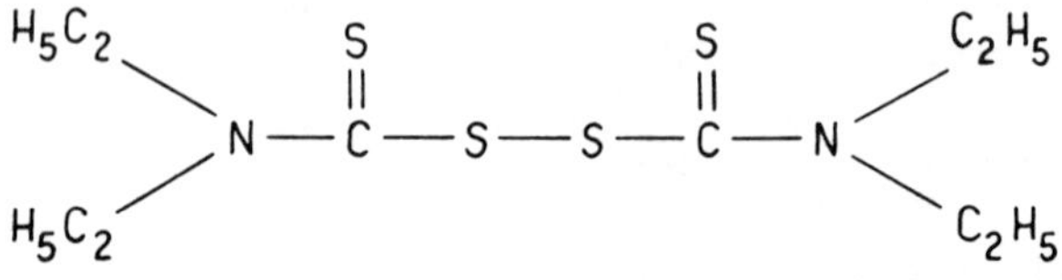

Structure II

Summary

1. Drug metabolism is a primary mechanism for removal of drugs from the body.

2. Drugs may undergo Phase I or Phase II metabolism depending on their structure.

3. The major site for drug metabolism is the microsomal fraction of the liver.

4. Drug metabolism may vary between species and may be affected by age. Sex differences in drug metabolism in humans are minor, and are not clinically important.

5. Metabolism can be induced and inhibited by various agents.

Literature Cited

1. Williams, R. T. *Detoxication Mechanisms;* Wiley: New York, 1959.
2. Creasey, W. A. *Drug Disposition in Humans;* Oxford University Press: New York, 1979.
3. Hildebrandt, A.; Estabrook, R. W. *Arch. Biochem. Biophys.*, **1977,** *143,* 66–79.
4. Goldstein, A.; Aranow, L.; Kalman, S. M. *Principles of Drug Action;* Harper and Row: New York, 1969.
5. LaDu, B. N.; Mandell, H. G.; Way, E. L.; Eds. *Fundamentals of Drug Metabolism and Drug Disposition;* Williams and Wilkins: Baltimore, 1971.
6. Gorrod, J. W.; Beckett, A. H. *Drug Metabolism in Man;* Taylor and Francis: London, 1978.
7. Jenner, P.; Testa, B. *Concepts in Drug Metabolism;* Marcel Dekker: New York, 1980.
8. Vesell, E.S. *Fed. Proc.* **1972,** *31,* 253–1269.
9. Ward, R. M; Singh, S.; Mirkin, B. L. *Fetal Clinical Pharmacology in Drug Treatment: Principles and Practices of Clinical Pharmacology and Therapeutics;* Avery, G. S., Ed.; ADIS: New York, 1980; pp 76–96.
10. Weiss, C. F.; Glazko, A. J.; Weston, J. K. *New Engl. J. Med.* **1960,** *262,* 787–794.

9

Renal Excretion

A number of nonrenal routes may contribute to removal of compounds from the body. For example, the lungs, saliva, sweat, direct excretion into the GI tract, and biliary excretion all remove compounds from the body. However, the major excretory pathway for most substances is provided by the kidneys. Even when a compound is extensively metabolized in the liver or elsewhere, the metabolites must be voided via the kidneys in most cases.

Human renal blood flow rate is about 1.2 L/min or 1730 L/day. This amount represents 25% of total cardiac output. Blood enters the kidneys via the renal arteries from the abdominal aorta, and leaves the kidneys via the renal veins to return to the general circulation via the inferior vena cava. The 1.2 L of blood that perfuses the kidneys each minute contains about 650 mL of plasma water. Of this plasma water, about 130 mL is filtered at the glomerulus. This filtration results in about 170–190 L of plasma water each day. Of this, approximately 1.5 L of fluid is excreted as urine each day, the remainder being absorbed back into the circulation. Thus, the kidneys receive a large proportion of the circulation, and they have developed very efficient methods to filter and secrete substances and to excrete them in a concentrated urine (1).

The functional unit of the kidney is the nephron (Figure 9.1), of which there are a million or more in each human kidney. From a pharmacokinetic viewpoint, the kidney can be considered to consist of five major components: the glomerulus (or Bowman's capsule), the proximal convoluted tubule, the loop of Henle, the distal convoluted tubule, and the collecting tubule and ducts.

0065-7719/86/0185-0121$06.00/1
© 1986 American Chemical Society

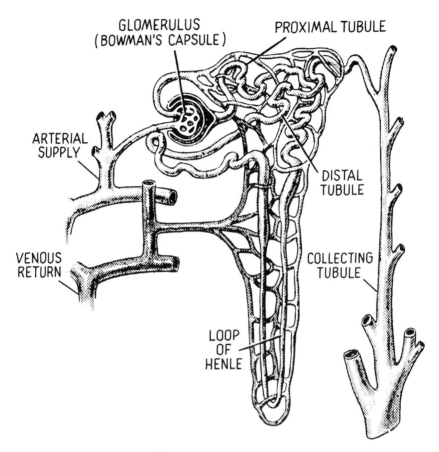

Figure 9.1. The functional nephron. (Reproduced with permission from Smith, H.W. The Kidney: Structure and Function in Health and Disease; Oxford University Press: New York; 1951.)

The glomerulus is concerned with filtration of plasma water and its contents into the tubule. This filtration is passive and relatively nonspecific because it is not influenced by fat solubility, ionization, or for the most part molecular size. An upper limit to molecular size exists because proteins, particularly soluble plasma proteins, are not filtered at the glomerulus. Therefore, any drug that is protein-bound cannot be filtered directly at the glomerulus.

The proximal tubule is concerned with reabsorption of sodium chloride and water. However, from a pharmacokinetic viewpoint, the most important function of the proximal tubule is active secretion of various drugs from the plasma via the capillaries adjacent to the nephron into the kidney tubule. This second mechanism of drug clearance from the body is more drug-specific than filtration. Secretion is an active, energy-consuming process, and different mechanisms exist for secreting acids (or anions) and bases (or cations), including quaternary ammonium compounds. Although drugs that are bound to plasma proteins cannot be actively secreted, the process of secretion is so rapid that bound drug may dissociate from protein and be secreted during a single pass through the kidney. Secretion may be so efficient that virtually all of the drug in blood may be removed in a single pass through the kidney, whether or not drug is bound to plasma proteins or even located in the red cells.

Henle's loop is a fine structure that passes from the renal cortex into the medulla and then returns to the cortex. This loop is concerned with sodium chloride and water reabsorption, but does not appear to play a major role in drug excretion.

In the distal tubules, acidification of urine (pH ~ 6) and further sodium chloride and water reabsorption occurs. However, the most important activity in the distal tubules with respect to the rate and efficiency of drug excretion is that of drug reabsorption. In some cases reabsorption may be an active process, for example, reabsorption of glucose and probenecid. But for the most part, reabsorption is passive and, like most other passive membrane-transport processes, favors un-ionized, fat-soluble compounds. The collecting ducts are concerned with water reabsorption and act under the control of the pituitary hormone vasopressin. Collecting ducts do not appear to play a major role in drug elimination (2,3).

From a pharmacokinetic viewpoint, each of the three major sites in the nephron is associated with a particular function related to drug excretion:

1. Passive filtration at the glomerulus, which is restricted to drug that is unbound to plasma proteins.

2. Active secretion at the proximal kidney tubule, which is essentially independent of protein binding but dependent upon molecular structure.

3. Passive reabsorption at the distal tubule, which is restricted to un-ionized, fat-soluble compounds.

Renal function can be determined by means of specific marker compounds. For example, creatinine, a substance that is produced in the body from muscle metabolism, and also inulin, a synthetic polymer hydrocarbon, are both filtered at the glomerulus, but are neither secreted nor reabsorbed in the tubules. Approximately 130 mL of plasma water is filtered by the kidneys, and is therefore efficiently cleared of creatinine and inulin (regardless of concentration) during each minute. Thus, the *plasma clearance* is equal to the glomerular filtration rate (GFR), which is approximately 130 mL/min.

Other compounds, for example, *p*-aminohippurate (PAH) and some penicillins and cephalosporins, are not only filtered at the glomerulus, but are also actively secreted at the proximal convoluted tubule. Because this process is very efficient, all of the drug may be removed from the blood or plasma during a single pass through the kidney, and the clearance (or the volume of plasma completely cleared of drug per unit time) is equal to the renal plasma flow, which is 650 mL/min. Thus, PAH is typically used to measure effective renal plasma flow (ERPF) or effective renal blood flow (ERBF).

Glucose is filtered at the glomerulus and is not secreted in the proximal tubule, but is normally completely reabsorbed at the distal tubule. Glucose clearance under normal circumstances is essentially zero. However, reabsorption of glucose is an active process, and there is a threshold to the reabsorption rate that may be exceeded in cases of glucose overload. For example, glucose may be passed in the urine in diabetes. Passive reabsorption, on the other hand, is not saturable, and the requirement of fat solubility for reabsorption to occur is the essence of the relationship between drug metabolism (producing a more water-soluble derivative) and renal excretion in removing substances from the body.

The semipermeable nature of the membranes of the distal tubule can be used to treat such conditions as drug overdose. For example, acidification of urine by administering ammonium chloride will tend to favor reabsorption of acidic drugs but will inhibit reabsorption of basic drugs that will be ionized at the acidic pH. On the other hand, basification of urine by administering sodium bicarbonate will tend to favor reabsorption of basic drugs but will inhibit reabsorption of acidic drugs that will be more ionized at the basic pH. Therefore, a useful approach in cases of drug overdose is to make the urine acidic for basic drugs and to make the urine alkaline for acidic drugs to facilitate their removal from the body. This approach may be used in conjunction with diuresis to increase renal excretion of compounds.

Although protein-bound drugs or metabolites may be actively secreted in the proximal tubules, these drugs will not filter at the glomerulus. If this is the case, why is it that protein-bound drugs that are not secreted do not stay in the blood for a very long time? The answer is that such drugs may be voided quite rapidly in urine because of the continuous nature of kidney perfusion by circulating blood. During a 1-min period in a healthy kidney, 130 mL of plasma water, out of a total renal plasma flow of 650 mL, will be filtered. Because this process is simple filtration, the concentration of unbound drug in the unfiltered plasma water does not change, and the bound–unbound drug equilibrium is not perturbed. No further drug will dissociate from protein. However, of the 130 mL of plasma water that is filtered each minute, approximately 128 mL is reabsorbed from the loop of Henle, distal tubule, and collecting ducts. If the water is reabsorbed and the filtered drug, or any portion of filtered drug, remains in the tubule because it cannot be reabsorbed, then the effective concentration of free drug in plasma will be reduced, and protein-bound drug will dissociate to retain the bound–unbound equilibrium. Thus, although the percentage of binding remains constant, as is normally the case, the concentration of total drug will continuously drop with each pass through the kidney until all the drug is eventually removed.

The terms *plasma clearance* and *renal clearance* must be differentiated. These terms are sometimes used interchangeably, but they describe two entirely different phenomena. The clearances considered so far have been renal clearances. Renal clearances describe the volume of plasma cleared of drug per unit time as a result of urinary excretion. Renal clearance is determined from the relationship between the amount of compound voided in urine during a given time and the mean concentration of compound in plasma during that time. Renal clearance can be calculated by Equation 9.1.

$$Cl_r = UV'/C \qquad (9.1)$$

where Cl_r is renal clearance, in milliliters of plasma per minute, U is the concentration of drug in urine, V' is urine flow rate, and C is the mean concentration of drug in plasma during the urine collection interval. The symbol V' is used to differentiate urine volume from the drug distribution volume V.

The numerator in Equation 9.1 represents the quantity of drug recovered in urine in units of mass per unit time. Dividing the numerator by the concentration, C, yields the renal clearance in units of volume per unit time. The volume referred to in the renal clearance is volume of plasma.

Ideally, the value of C is held constant during the entire urine collection interval, and this constant value may be achieved by using an endogenous substance such as creatinine, or by continuous infusion of an exogenous marker substance such as inulin.

Clearance may also be calculated during a period of changing plasma levels, for example, following bolus intravenous injection of a drug. This method of clearance calculation is frequently done out of sheer necessity, but it may yield unreliable values because of bladder holdup, changing tissue distribution during the collection interval, and various other factors. Clearances should be measured several times through use of sequential urine collection intervals, and the results should be averaged to provide a best estimate.

To determine plasma clearance, a model must be proposed that differentiates between drug voided in urine and drug eliminated by other routes. A typical situation is one in which drug is removed from the body both by urinary excretion of unchanged drug and by hepatic metabolism. If both phenomena are nonsaturable and therefore first-order in nature, then first-order rate constants k_e and k_m can be assigned to urinary excretion of unchanged drug, and drug metabolism, respectively. If the arithmetic sum of k_e and k_m equals k_{el}, which is the rate constant for loss of drug from plasma by all elimination routes, then the model for drug loss can be shown as in Scheme 9.1. By using this model, the rate of drug loss from the body due to both urinary excretion and metabolism can be predicted by Equation 9.2, and the rate of drug loss due to urinary excretion alone can be predicted from Equation 9.3.

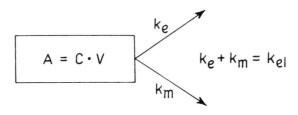

Scheme 9.1. Model for loss of drug from plasma by urinary excretion and metabolism. k_e is the first-order rate constant for urinary excretion of unchanged drug; k_m is the first-order rate constant for drug metabolism; k_{el} is the sum of k_e and k_m; A is the amount of drug in the body at any time t; C is the concentration of drug in plasma at any time t; V is the distribution volume of the drug in the body.

$$-[dA/dt_{(total)}] = k_{el}A = k_{el}CV \qquad (9.2)$$

$$-[dA/dt_{(renal)}] = K_eA = K_eCV \qquad (9.3)$$

Comparing Equations 9.1 and 9.3 yields Equation 9.4.

$$k_eCV = UV' \qquad (9.4)$$

Dividing both sides of Equation 9.4 by the plasma concentration term C yields Equation 9.5.

$$k_eV = UV'/C \qquad (9.5)$$

This equation provides an expression for the renal clearance, UV'/C, in terms of the first-order urinary excretion constant, k_e, and the drug distribution volume in the body, V. However, the term k_eV describes only the fraction of plasma clearance due to renal excretion. If the drug is not metabolized and is eliminated entirely as unchanged drug, then $k_m = 0$ because no metabolism occurs, $k_{el} = k_e$, and Equation 9.5 can be rewritten as Equation 9.6.

$$k_{el}V = UV'/C = Cl_p \qquad (9.6)$$

However, if metabolism or any other nonrenal elimination pathway occurs, then $k_{el} > k_e$, because of the contribution of k_m, and the true plasma clearance $k_{el}V$ will be greater than the renal clearance, UV'/C.

Thus renal clearance, which is due to the renal elimination of unchanged drug, is distinguished from plasma clearance, which is due to all elimination processes. Metabolism clearance, frequently called hepatic clearance, can similarly be described using the product k_mV. Clearance by other organs can also be described simply by substituting the appropriate rate constant. However, the total plasma clearance, $k_{el}V$, will always be equal to or greater than the renal clearance, or any other organ clearance.

Another factor often complicates accurate interpretation of clearance values. Both Equations 9.1 and 9.2 contain the term C, which represents the concentration of drug in plasma. Because drugs bind to plasma proteins to varying degrees, the question arises as to whether the value of C should represent the concentration of total drug or the concentration of free drug. In other words, should the clearance value be uncorrected, or should the clearance value be corrected for plasma-protein binding?

This question is difficult to answer because the clearance depends on the precise mechanism for drug elimination, and the mechanism is frequently unknown. For example, if a drug has a renal clearance of 130 mL/min, this value could arise because the drug is removed from the plasma solely by glomerular filtration, in which case protein-bound drug plays no part in the elimination process, or because the drug is actively secreted in the proximal tubules but subsequently partially reabsorbed at the distal tubules, in which case protein-bound drug does play a role in the elimination process. If the actual mechanism of elimination can be defined, then a reasonable rule of thumb is that if protein-bound drug does not participate in the elimination process, then the corrected clearance should be used. In other words, the unbound drug goes into the denominator of Equation 9.1 and into the right side of Equation 9.2. On the other hand, if protein-bound drug does participate in the elimination process, then the uncorrected clearance should be used, and the concentration of total drug should be used in the equations.

Relationship Among Clearance, Drug Elimination Rate, and Half-Life

By definition, the biological or *plasma half-life* of a drug is the time taken for drug concentration in plasma to be reduced by one-half. In all first-order processes, the half-life is a constant and is related to the first-order rate constant as in Equation 9.7.

$$t_{1/2} = \ln 2/k = 0.693/k \qquad (9.7)$$

Thus, if a drug has an elimination half-life of 1 h, then the drug concentration in plasma will be reduced by one-half each hour. If, at time 0, the concentration is 100 μg/mL, then at 1 h the concentration will be reduced to 50 μg/mL, at 2 h to 25 μg/mL, and at 3 h to 12.5 μg/mL.

A relationship between drug clearance and half-life can be established from Equation 9.7. By combining Equations 9.6 and 9.7, Equation 9.8 is obtained, which rearranges to Equation 9.9.

$$Cl_p = 0.693V/t_{1/2} \qquad (9.8)$$

$$t_{1/2} = 0.693V/Cl_p \qquad (9.9)$$

This equation shows that the half-life of a drug is directly related to the drug distribution volume, but inversely related to drug clearance. The effect that volume has on drug elimination rate or half-life for a given clearance is demonstrated in Figure 9.2.

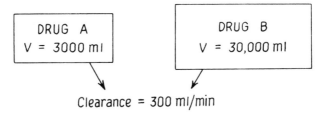

Clearance = 300 ml/min

(A) 10% of volume cleared of drug each minute.
(B) 1% of volume cleared of drug each minute.

Figure 9.2. Relationship between distribution volume, clearance, and elimination rate.

In this figure, Drug A distributes into a volume of 3 L and Drug B distributes into a 10-fold greater volume of 30 L. Although the clearance of the two drugs is identical, 10% of the total body load of Drug A is cleared during 1 min, compared to only 1% of Drug B. Therefore, the elimination rate of Drug A will be 10 times greater than that of Drug B, and the elimination half-life of Drug A will be 10 times shorter than that of Drug B, despite an identical clearance value. This relationship can be summarized by noting that clearance describes an intrinsic ability of an organ or organ system to remove drug from the body. Clearance is completely independent of drug distribution volume. On the other hand, the half-life, or the elimination rate constant, is a complex function of both the clearance and the distribution volume of a drug or its metabolites. Although Equation 9.6 might be interpreted as inferring a relationship between volume and clearance, this interpretation is not the case. Any change in volume would result in a change in the elimination rate constant, not the clearance. These interesting relationships are summarized in Table 9.1. For a given clearance, the half-life of a drug increases with increasing distribution volume, and for a given distribution volume, the half-life decreases with increasing clearance. The shortest drug half-life is obtained with a drug that has a high clearance and a small distribution volume. The longest half-life is obtained with a drug that has a low clearance and a large distribution volume.

Table 9.1—Influence of Distribution Volume on Drug Half-Life

	Drug Half-Life in Plasma (h)		
Cl_p	$V = 5\ L$	$V = 25\ L$	$V = 100\ L$
50 mL/min (reabsorption)	1.2	5.8	23.1
130 mg/min (filtration)	0.4	2.2	8.9
650 mL/min (secretion)	0.09	0.44	1.8

NOTE: Cl_p denotes plasma clearance.

Renal Disease

All of the relationships just described are based on normally functioning kidneys. Most compounds, whether drug or metabolite, are eventually cleared via the kidneys. If kidney function becomes impaired, the kidneys lose the ability to eliminate substances to varying degrees. When considering the possible impact of impaired renal function on drug or metabolite clearance, and the necessity of dose adjustment in this condition, a number of questions must be answered. These questions are (1) is the drug cleared by the kidneys, (2) are its metabolites cleared by the kidneys, (3) are the metabolites pharmacologically active, and (4) how much excess accumulation of drug, metabolite, or both can be tolerated before the dose has to be modified to avoid toxic side effects? Much has been written on this subject (4,5). Space permits description only of some basic concepts associated with drug disposition and dosage in renal failure, and some of the unresolved problems in this area of research.

Renal failure can result from a variety of pathological conditions. If impairment of renal function is rapid in onset and of relatively short duration, then the renal failure is described as acute. The primary cause of this condition may be acute congestive heart failure, shock, acute tubular necrosis, or hypercalcemia. The condition is generally reversible, although complete restoration of renal function may take from 6 to 12 months.

Chronic renal failure is distinguished from the acute condition because chronic renal failure is almost always caused by intrinsic renal disease and is characterized by slow, progressive development. Unlike the acute condition, chronic renal impairment is generally irreversible. The degree of loss of kidney functional capacity in the chronic condition is best described in terms of the *intact nephron hypothesis,* which considers that the diseased kidney comprises normal nephrons and nephrons that are essentially nonfunctional due to the pathological condition. Progressive impairment of renal function is reflected in an increased fraction of nonfunctional nephrons.

The prolonged and progressive nature of chronic renal failure is of particular concern in elderly patients who may require a variety of medications. The inability of these patients to excrete drugs and drug metabolites adequately, and the influence of their uremic condition on the function of other physiological systems, requires careful drug dosage adjustment to achieve adequate therapeutic blood and urine concentrations without toxicity. Some common causes of kidney failure are given in Table 9.2.

Table 9.2—Some Common Causes of Kidney Failure

Cause	Description
Pyelonephritis	Inflammation and deterioration of the pyelonephrons due to infection, antigens, or other idiopathic causes.
Hypertension	Chronic overloading of the kidney with fluid and electrolytes may lead to kidney insufficiency.
Diabetes mellitus	Disturbance of sugar metabolism and acid–base balance may lead to or predispose a patient to degenerative renal disease.
Nephrotoxic drugs or metals	Certain drugs taken chronically may cause irreversible kidney damage, e.g., the aminoglycosides, phenacetin, and heavy metals such as mercury and lead.
Hypovolemia	Any condition that causes a reduction in renal blood flow will eventually lead to renal ischemia and damage.

SOURCE: Reproduced with permission from reference 5. Copyright 1980, Appleton-Century-Crofts.

Methods of Measuring Renal Function

Renal function can be measured in several ways. The most common method involves determining circulating levels and excretion of creatinine, or creatinine clearance. Creatinine is formed from muscle metabolism in the body and circulates in the plasma of individuals with normal renal function at a concentration of approximately 1 mg%. Creatinine is cleared via the kidneys by filtration to yield the familiar creatinine clearance of about 130 mL/min. This value depends partially on body size, degree of activity, muscle mass, and age. Various nomographs have been described to account for these.

As kidney function declines, for whatever reason, the glomerular filtration rate, and hence the creatinine clearance, will also decline. If the kidneys are working with only 50% efficiency, the creatinine clearance will drop to 50 or 60 mL/min, depending on age and other factors. According to the intact nephron hypothesis, other kidney functions will also decline, including tubular secretion. This decline in kidney function leads to the reasonable assumption that, provided a compound is cleared via the kidney, clearance will be affected to a similar extent as creatinine clearance, even though the compound may be filtered and secreted, or filtered, secreted, and also reabsorbed!

Creatinine clearance, like any other renal clearance value, is generally calculated from the relationship in Equation 9.10.

$$Cl_{cr} = \frac{\text{rate of urinary excretion of creatinine}}{\text{serum concentration of creatinine}} \qquad (9.10)$$

Numerical values are substituted into this equation to show a normal creatinine clearance of 130 mL/min in Equation 9.11.

$$Cl_{cr} = (1.3 \text{ mg/min})/(0.01 \text{ mg/mL}) = 130 \text{ mL/min} \qquad (9.11)$$

Several methods have been described by which creatinine clearance can be used to predict the effect of renal function impairment on drug elimination. One method of general application is described in Equation 9.12.

$$k = k_{nr} + XCl_{cr} \qquad (9.12)$$

where k is the drug elimination rate constant in reciprocal hours, k_{nr} is the drug elimination rate constant with zero kidney function in reciprocal hours, Cl_{cr} is the creatinine clearance in milliliters per minute, and X is a constant.

Suppose that a drug is cleared entirely via the kidneys. When creatinine clearance reduces to zero, in the case of complete renal impairment, k will become zero because k_{nr} is zero. Consider, on the other hand, a drug that is cleared in equal proportions by the kidneys and by the liver (metabolism or biliary excretion). Then in complete renal shutdown, the value of k will reduce to k_{nr}, which is one-half the value of k in a normal individual, and the elimination rate in complete renal failure is one-half the normal value. Thus, if the elimination rate of a drug under normal conditions, the amount of drug cleared by the kidneys, and the amount of drug cleared by other processes are known, then the extent to which drug elimination will be impaired in declining renal function can be predicted with reasonable accuracy.

Some drugs for which this information is available are given in Table 9.3, and the relationships between creatinine clearance and decrease in elimination rate for each of the drug groups is illustrated in Figure 9.3 (4). The changes in drug half-life are shown on the right side of the figure. From Table 9.3 and Figure 9.3, drugs in Group A, which include minocycline, rifampicin, lidocaine, and digitoxin, are shown to be cleared to a very small extent by the kidneys in normal individuals. Elimination of these drugs is therefore not influenced by renal function, and dosage adjustment in renal impairment is not necessary. Drugs in Group L, on the other hand, are handled almost exclusively by the kidneys. Elimination is markedly impaired with declining renal function, and dosage adjustment in renal impairment is likely to be mandatory.

Methods of Dosage Adjustment

Many options and opinions exist as to the optimal way to adjust the drug dosage in renally compromised patients, but all options have the common objective of reducing the drug dosage to maintain therapeutic drug levels and avoid undue accumulation. In essence, drug input has to be reduced to the same extent that drug elimination is reduced by renal function impairment.

The following two alternatives form the basis of most methods. The first alternative is to reduce the drug dose size, but maintain the same dosage interval as in normal renal function. The degree of dose reduction is given in Equation 9.13.

$$\text{uremic dose} = \text{normal dose}\ (k_u/k_n) \tag{9.13}$$

where k_u and k_n are, respectively, drug elimination rate constants in uremic and normal individuals. The dose is reduced according to the ratio of the observed k in the uremic individual to that in a normal person. If k is halved, then the dose must also be reduced by one-half.

The second alternative is given in Equation 9.14.

$$\text{uremic dosage interval} = \text{normal dosage interval}\ (t_{1/2u}/t_{1/2n}) \tag{9.14}$$

The dosing interval must be increased according to the increase in elim-

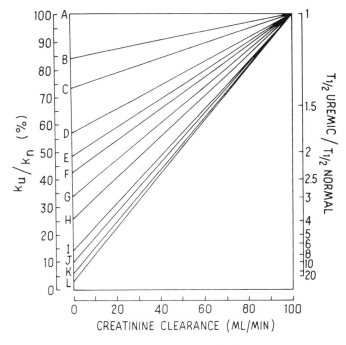

Figure 9.3. Changes in the percentage of normal elimination rate constant (left ordinate), and the consequent geometric increase in elimination half-life (right ordinate), as a function of creatinine clearance. (Reproduced with permission from reference 6. Copyright 1976, American Pharmaceutical Association.)

ination half-life in the uremic patient while giving the same quantity of drug in each dose to that given to a normal patient.

Application of these two approaches for gentamicin in a patient with a creatinine clearance of 10 mL/min is shown in Figure 9.4. Although both methods yield the same mean serum level, the shapes of the serum drug profiles are quite different. Regardless of the method of dosage adjustment, achieving an identical drug blood profile in a uremic patient to that in a normal individual is impossible.

The relative merits of the two approaches are argued but have not been resolved. The decision to adjust drug dosage at all in renal impairment depends on the type of drug. For example, most penicillins and cephalosporins have wide therapeutic indices, are relatively nontoxic, and generally do not require dose adjustment, except in cases of severe impairment. The aminoglycosides, on the other hand, are potentially highly toxic, and dosage has to be carefully titrated to renal function.

The previous discussion has provided only a brief glimpse at some pharmacokinetic aspects of the clinical problem of dosage adjustment in

Table 9.3—Elimination Rate Constants for Various Drugs

Group	Drug	$k_n(h^{-1})$	$k_{nr}(h^{-1})$	$k_{nr}/k_n(\%)$
A	Minocycline	0.04	0.04	100.0
	Rifampicin	0.25	0.25	100.0
	Lidocaine	0.39	0.36	92.3
	Digitoxin	0.114	0.10	87.7
B	Doxycycline	0.037	0.031	83.3
	Chlortetracycline	0.12	0.095	79.2
C	Clindamycin	0.16	0.12	75.0
	Chloramphenicol	0.26	0.19	73.1
	Propranolol	0.22	0.16	72.8
	Erythromycin	0.39	0.28	71.8
D	Trimethoprim	0.054	0.031	57.4
	Isoniazid (fast)	0.53	0.30	56.6
	Isoniazid (slow)	0.23	0.13	56.5
E	Dicloxacillin	1.20	0.60	50.0
	Sulfadiazine	0.069	0.032	46.4
	Sulfamethoxazole	0.084	0.037	44.0
F	Nafcillin	1.26	0.54	42.8
	Chlorpropamide	0.020	0.008	40.0
	Lincomycin	0.15	0.06	40.0
G	Colistimethate	0.154	0.054	35.1
	Oxacillin	1.73	0.58	33.6
	Digoxin	0.021	0.07	33.3
H	Tetracycline	0.120	0.033	27.5
	Cloxacillin	1.21	0.31	25.6
	Oxytetracycline	0.075	0.014	18.7
I	Amoxicillin	0.70	0.10	14.3
	Methicillin	1.40	0.19	13.6
J	Ticarcillin	0.58	0.066	11.4
	Penicillin G	1.24	0.13	10.5
K	Cefazolin	0.32	0.02	6.2
	Cephaloridine	0.51	0.03	5.9
	Cephalothin	1.20	0.06	5.0
	Gentamicin	0.30	0.015	5.0
L	Flucytosine	0.18	0.007	3.9
	Kanamycin	0.28	0.01	3.6
	Vancomycin	0.12	0.004	3.3
	Tobramycin	0.32	0.010	3.1
	Cephalexin	1.54	0.032	2.1

renal failure. Many other aspects that confound the task of providing useful, nontoxic therapy to uremic individuals have not been discussed. Similarly, the important problems of altered distribution and protein binding in renal failure, the use of serum creatinine, and conversion of serum creatinine values to creatinine clearance for renal function estimation are not covered here but are described in detail elsewhere (4,5).

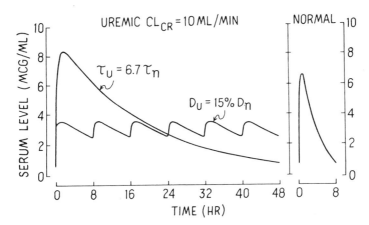

Figure 9.4. Predicted steady-state serum levels of gentamicin in a 70-kg normal subject and in a patient with a creatinine clearance of 10 mL/min. The dose D_n, dosing interval τ, and elimination rate constant k_n in normal renal function are 1.7 mg/kg, 8 h, and 0.347 h^{-1}, respectively. V_n is 14 L and is assumed to be unchanged in renal failure. Adjusted doses and dosage intervals for the uremic patient are obtained from Figure 9.3.

Summary

1. Drug elimination via the kidneys involves three different processes: glomerular filtration, proximal tubule secretion, and distal tubule reabsorption.

2. Drugs may be subject to one or more of these processes depending on their protein binding, molecular structure, and fat solubility.

3. Plasma clearance may be equal to or greater than renal clearance. Both of these phenomena may be calculated in corrected or uncorrected form depending on the mechanism of elimination and the degree of dependence on protein binding.

4. Drug half-life is related to clearance but is influenced also by distribution volume. Clearance, on the other hand, is independent of distribution volume and describes an intrinsic relationship between a substance and the eliminating organ or organ systems.

5. Drug elimination may be markedly affected by renal function impairment depending on the fraction of drug that is cleared by the kidneys. Dosage adjustment may be necessary to avoid toxic overdose, depending on the degree of impairment and the therapeutic index of the drug.

Literature Cited

1. Giusti, D. L. In *Clinical Pharmacy and Therapeutics*; Hirschman, J. I.; Herfindal, E. T.; Eds.; Williams and Wilkins: 1925; pp 69–79.

2. Weiner, I. M. *Ann. Rev. Pharmacol.* **1967,** *7,* 39–56.
3. Cafruny, E. J. *Ann. Rev. Pharmacol.* **1968,** *8,* 131–150.
4. Welling, P. G.; Craig, W. A. In *The Effects of Disease States on Drug Pharmacokinetics;* Benet, L. Z., Ed.; American Pharmaceutical Association: Washington, DC; 1976, pp 155–187.
5. Shargel, L.; Yu, A. B. C. *Applied Biopharmaceutics and Pharmacokinetics;* Appleton-Century-Crofts: New York, 1980, pp 102–115, 187–203.

Problems

1. During intravenous infusion therapy, urinary recovery of unchanged drug averaged 180 mg/h during three consecutive 1-h collection intervals. The plasma drug level during the entire 3-h period was a constant value of 10 μg/mL. Calculate the renal clearance of unchanged drug in units of milliliters per minute.

2. Urinary recovery of unchanged drug in Problem 1 accounted for one-half of the loss of drug from the body by all routes. What is the plasma clearance?

3. If the true distribution volume of the drug in Problem 2 is 42 L, then what is the elimination half-life of the drug in plasma?

4. A drug is cleared from plasma via the kidneys by a combination of glomerular filtration and active tubular secretion with some distal tubular reabsorption. If the drug is highly bound to plasma proteins, should the plasma clearance be corrected for protein binding?

THE MATHEMATICS
OF PHARMACOKINETICS

10

The One-Compartment Open Model with Intravenous Dosage

To understand the mathematical approach used throughout this book, a basic knowledge of calculus is needed. Initially some kinetic expressions will be derived. However, with some exceptions, mathematical derivation will be kept to a minimum. Helpful integrating procedures, such as the Laplace transform, must be used to solve rate equations for complex pharmacokinetic expressions. However, the intent of this book is not to teach mathematics but to provide a basic understanding of pharmacokinetics and its uses. Therefore, only minor emphasis will be placed on derivations, and major emphasis will be placed on the meaning, use, and application of pharmacokinetic principles.

Drug input, elimination, and transfer between pharmacokinetic compartments will be assumed to be first-order and linear. This assumption is consistent with the modeling approach. In later chapters, departures from this general approach will be described, but the principal arguments will be developed assuming first-order, nonsaturable, and either reversible kinetics (e.g., between spatial compartments) or irreversible (e.g., between chemical compartments, and also absorption and elimination).

To reiterate a comment in Chapter 1, the pharmacokinetic compartment can be used to describe both spatial and chemical states. For example, if a drug appears to distribute in a heterogeneous manner in the

0065-7719/86/0185-0139$07.00/1
© 1986 American Chemical Society

body so that overall drug distribution can be described in terms of two distinct body volumes, then the concentration of drug in these volumes and its distribution between them are described in terms of two spatial compartments. On the other hand, if a drug forms a metabolite, particularly if the metabolite is active, which makes it of interest, then the metabolite is considered to be a separate chemical compartment, regardless of whether the metabolite occupies the same or different body fluids and tissues as the parent drug. Spatial and chemical compartments can coexist in the same kinetic model. For any drug that is metabolized, coexistence is necessarily the case.

Consider the simplest model of all, the one-compartment open model. Despite its associated simplifications and assumptions, this model is the most common for describing drug profiles in blood, plasma, serum, or urine after oral or intramuscular doses. Following intravenous bolus doses, an additional drug distribution phase is often more readily discernable. This situation will be discussed in more detail later. In the simple one-compartment model, however, the drug is assumed to rapidly distribute into a homogeneous fluid volume in the body regardless of the route of administration (1, 2).

Pharmacokinetic rate constants are based on transfer of amounts of drugs. Rate constants are applied to concentration changes subsequently by dividing the expressions by the appropriate distribution volumes. Also, on a microscopic basis, most pharmacokinetic rate constants describe a multiplicity of events. For example, an absorption rate constant is possibly influenced by dissolution, stomach emptying, splanchnic blood flow, and a variety of other factors. However, despite the gross simplification involved, observed rate constants describe the overall rate-limiting process, be it absorption, distribution, metabolism, or excretion. How much more mechanistic information can be obtained from such rate constants depends on the drug and the enthusiasm and ingenuity of the investigator.

The One-Compartment Open Model with Bolus Intravenous Injection

This model is depicted in Scheme 10.1. The box, or compartment, represents the drug distribution volume, and other values and rate constants are defined in the caption. The value k_{el} is equal to the sum of all elimination rate constants, including those for drug eliminated via sweat, bile, lungs, etc. However, in this example only two routes of elimination are assumed, urinary excretion and metabolism. The curved arrow leading into the compartment represents instantaneous introduction of drug.

Using this model, Equation 10.1 can be written in the following form.

$$dA/dt = -(k_e + k_m)A = -k_{el}A \qquad (10.1)$$

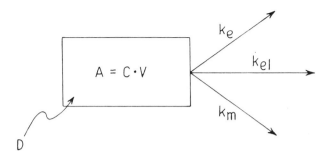

Scheme 10.1. One-compartment open model with bolus intravenous injection: D is the dose, A is the amount of drug in the body, and C is the concentration of drug in body fluids.

where A is the amount of drug in the body, t is time, k_e is the rate constant for urinary excretion, and k_m is the rate constant for metabolism. Equation 10.1 describes the rate of loss of drug from the body. This equation rearranges to

$$dA/A = -k_{el}\,dt \tag{10.2}$$

Equation 10.2, when integrated between the limits of zero and finite time, when the value A varying from A_0, the initial amount of drug in the body, to some value less than A_0, becomes

$$\ln A - \ln A_0 = -k_{el}t \tag{10.3}$$

The natural logarithms appear in this expression because the integral of the reciprocal of any single value X is equal to the natural logarithm of X. Rearrangement of Equation 10.3 yields

$$\ln (A/A_0) = -k_{el}t \tag{10.4}$$

If both sides of Equation 10.4 are made into a power of e, as in Equation 10.5, Equation 10.6 is obtained.

$$e^{\ln (A/A_0)} = e^{-k_{el}t} \tag{10.5}$$

$$A/A_0 = e^{-k_{el}t} \quad \text{or} \quad A = A_0\,e^{-k_{el}t} \tag{10.6}$$

Equation 10.5 converts to Equation 10.6 because e to the power of the natural logarithm of X is equal to X ($e^{\ln X} = X$). This is analogous to logarithms to the base 10. To use a numerical example, the logarithm to the base 10 of 100 is equal to 2, and 10^2 is 100. Thus, 10 raised to the power of the logarithm of 100 is equal to 100, or 10 raised to the power of the logarithm X is equal to X.

Equation 10.6 can be converted into concentration terms by dividing both sides of the expression by V, the distribution volume, as in Equation 10.7, to yield Equation 10.8.

$$A/V = (A_0/V)\, e^{-k_{el}t} \tag{10.7}$$

$$C = C_0 e^{-k_{el}t} \tag{10.8}$$

where C is the concentration of drug in the body, and C_0 is the concentration of drug initially. Equation 10.3 can similarly be converted to concentration form as in

$$\ln C = \ln C_0 - k_{el}t \quad \text{or} \quad \log C = \log C_0 - k_{el}t/2.3 \tag{10.9}$$

The conversion from natural logarithms to logarithms to the base 10 in Equation 10.9 is obtained from the simple relationship that $\ln X = 2.3 \log X$.

What information can be obtained about a drug by using some of these expressions? From Equations 10.8 and 10.9, a plot of the logarithm of the drug concentration against time will be linear. Logarithms to the base 10 will be used in this book because logarithmic graph paper is printed that way, and it is thus more convenient.

In Figure 10.1, the slope of the line, which will be linear if the data fit the model, gives the elimination rate constant k_{el}, and the extrapolated intercept at time zero gives C_0. Actually, the intercept is the logarithm of C_0, but as the actual concentration values are plotted on semilogarithmic

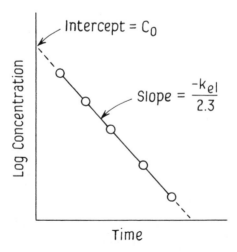

Figure 10.1. Plot of logarithm of drug concentration versus time following intravenous bolus injection.

graph paper, the paper is converting actual values into logarithmic values. Actual concentration values can therefore be read directly from the plots.

The overall elimination half-life of the drug can also be obtained from the relationship in Equation 10.10.

$$t_{1/2} = \ln 2/k_{el} = 0.693/k_{el} \tag{10.10}$$

Equation 10.10 is valid for any first-order rate constant. However, instead of finding the elimination rate constant and then calculating the half-life, obtaining these values in reverse order is usually more convenient when analyzing data graphically. For example, the elimination half-life can be obtained by selecting any time interval during which the value of C is reduced by one-half. Whichever values of C are used, the time interval for C to reduce by half will be the same. The value of k_{el} is then obtained from Equation 10.10.

If the administered dose D is divided by the extrapolated value C_0, and if the reasonable assumption is made that all of the injected dose was absorbed, then the drug distribution volume is obtained from

$$V = D/C_0 \tag{10.11}$$

A word of caution is appropriate here. During this and subsequent exercises, the simplifying assumption is made that drugs are not bound, or are bound to only a negligible extent, to plasma and tissue proteins or other macromolecules. This assumption saves considerable time and keeps the mathematics relatively simple. However, if binding does occur, then appropriate adjustments may be made to such parameters as distribution volume, which was described previously.

The drug elimination half-life, overall elimination rate constant k_{el}, and its distribution volume have now been calculated from the data in Figure 10.1. Multiplying the distribution volume V by the elimination rate constant k_{el}, as in Equation 10.12, yields the plasma clearance, Cl_p.

$$Cl_p = Vk_{el} \tag{10.12}$$

Knowing also the renal clearance and differentiating it from other clearance processes would be useful information. This information cannot be obtained from plasma data alone because the information in Figure 10.1 indicates only how rapidly the drug is leaving the body. The figure provides no information regarding the route of elimination. However, if all of the drug that is excreted in unchanged form in the urine, A_u^∞, were collected, then the renal clearance can be obtained from

$$Cl_r/Cl_p = k_e V/k_{el} V = k_e/k_{el} = A_u^\infty/D \tag{10.13}$$

where Cl_p is the plasma clearance, Cl_r is the renal clearance, and A_u^∞ is the amount of drug excreted in urine.

The renal clearance is thus related to plasma clearance in direct proportion to the ratio of total urinary recovery of unchanged drug to the administered dose. As discussed previously, renal clearance may be equal to or less than plasma clearance, but never greater. That is, k_e can never be greater than k_{el}. Once k_e is obtained, k_m can be calculated simply by subtracting k_e from k_{el}, as in Equation 10.14.

$$k_m = k_{el} - k_e \qquad (10.14)$$

Another useful pharmacokinetic parameter that can be obtained from intravenous data, or from any other data for that part, is the area under the plasma level curve, AUC.

The total area under the plasma curve, that is, the area from zero to infinite time, is obtained mathematically by integrating the terms in Equation 10.8 between zero and infinite time. This integration, after appropriate cancellations, yields

$$AUC^{0\to\infty} = \int_0^\infty C = C_0 \int_0^\infty e^{-k_{el}t}\, dt$$

$$= -\frac{C_0}{k_{el}} (e^{-k_{el}\infty} - e^{-k_{el}0})$$

$$= -\frac{C_0}{k_{el}} (0 - 1) = \frac{C_0}{k_{el}} \qquad (10.15)$$

Because C_0 can be expressed as D/V, Equation 10.15 can be written as Equation 10.16.

$$AUC^{0\to\infty} = D/Vk_{el} = D/Cl_p \qquad (10.16)$$

This expression shows that the area under the plasma curve is equal to the dose divided by the plasma clearance. Perhaps more importantly, the plasma clearance can be obtained by dividing the dose by the area under the curve. However, the area must be the total area. If a truncated area is used, and this is frequently all that can be determined by direct observation of the data, an overestimation of the plasma clearance will result.

Renal clearance can also be determined with this approach, provided that the urinary recovery of unchanged drug is known. Renal clearance is readily obtained from

$$Cl_r = A_u t / AUC^{0\to t} \qquad (10.17)$$

Equation 10.17 is analogous to a rearranged form of Equation 10.16. Thus, renal clearance is calculated by dividing the quantity of drug recovered in urine up to a certain time by the area under the plasma curve up to the same time. (This time can be infinity but need not be.) The calculation for renal clearance has the advantage over calculation for plasma clearance because truncated areas and partial urine collections can be used. If the values in Equation 10.17 were extrapolated to infinity, then Equation 10.18 results.

$$Cl_r = A_u^\infty / AUC^{0 \to \infty} \tag{10.18}$$

Equation 10.8 shows that renal clearance and plasma clearance differ only in terms of the difference between the administered dose and urinary recovery of unchanged drug A_u^∞.

The Trapezoidal Rule

Equations 10.15 and 10.16 describe the area under the plasma curve following bolus intravenous injection. In many cases, however, area values are measured directly from the data, for example, in model-independent kinetics, and several methods are available to do this. These methods include planimetry, which is drawing the plasma profile on regular graph paper, cutting out the profile, and weighing the paper; the trapezoidal rule; and the log trapezoidal rule. The simple trapezoidal rule is described here because it is the most commonly used method. The trapezoidal rule is quick and accurate. The accuracy of the method is directly related to the number of data points.

A trapezoid is a four-sided figure with two sides parallel and two sides nonparallel. When the length of one of the sides is reduced to zero, the trapezoid becomes a triangle. If plasma data are plotted on regular graph paper, the area under the plasma profile can be divided into a series of trapezoids, and the areas of the individual trapezoids can be calculated and summed.

The data in Table 10.1 constitute a typical drug profile that might be obtained following bolus intravenous injection of a drug that has a biological half-life of 1 h. If these data were plotted on regular graph paper, and if the data points were joined by straight lines, a series of trapezoids would be obtained, terminating with a triangle for the 8–12-h interval. Calculating the area for each segment of the curve and cumulatively adding each successive segment yields the trapezoidal area in the third column of the table. In this example, the sampling time has been extended to when no detectable drug remains in the plasma. Unfortunately, this situation does not usually occur in practice. In most cases, the plasma sampling time is not extended for a sufficiently long period to allow plasma drug levels to decline to zero, so that the area calculated by the trapezoidal rule is the area from time zero to some time t when drug levels are still present. Thus, a truncated area is obtained, as in Figure 10.2. The 6-h plasma sample still contains drug, so the total area under the plasma level curve cannot be calculated.

The truncated area is useful for many types of calculations, but the complete area under the curve is more useful. For example, the area from time zero to infinity is required to calculate plasma clearance and total absorption and to construct Wagner–Nelson absorption plots, which will be discussed shortly. So, to be able to extend the truncated area to the area to infinite time is important.

The simplest and most common method to achieve this is by end correction. This method involves calculating the area from the last sampling time, C_t, to time infinity and adding this value to the truncated area. To calculate the terminal area from time t to infinity, this portion of the drug profile is treated as if it were a separate profile where $C_0 = C_t$. Then, just as the area to time infinity for the total curve can be calculated by Equation 10.15, the terminal area can be calculated by dividing C_t by k_{el}, as in

$$\text{AUC}^{t\to\infty} = C_t/k_{el} \tag{10.19}$$

Adding this calculated area to the truncated area obtained by the trapezoidal rule will yield the area from zero to infinite time. End correction has been used here to correct or complete an area following intravenous

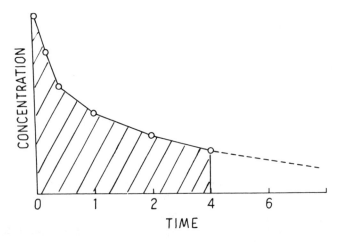

Figure 10.2. Truncated area under the drug concentration versus time curve in plasma.

Table 10.1—A Typical Drug Profile Following Bolus IV
Injection

Time (h)	Concentration ($\mu g/mL$)	Cumulative AUC ($\mu g \cdot h/mL$)
0	25.0	
0.25	21.0	5.75
0.50	17.6	10.58
1.0	12.5	18.11
2.0	6.25	27.49
3.0	3.13	32.18
4.0	1.56	34.53
6.0	0.40	36.49
8.0	0.10	36.99
12.0	0.0	37.19

dosing. However, end correction can be used equally well after any route of administration by following any drug profile, provided drug concentrations have been taken for sufficient time to identify and characterize the elimination rate constant k_{el}.

Regarding the data in Table 10.1, suppose that the sampling time had not been extended beyond 4 h so that the trapezoidal area also extended to 4 h. How would the end correction be calculated to obtain the total area from zero to infinite time?

The first step is to plot the data on semilogarithmic graph paper to obtain the linear descending portion of the drug concentration in plasma profile, and thereby calculate the drug half-life and elimination rate constant. Then by substituting the appropriate values into Equation 10.19, Equation 10.20 is obtained.

$$\text{AUC}^{4\to\infty} = C_t/k_{el} = 1.56/0.693 = 2.25 \ \mu g \cdot h/mL \quad (10.20)$$

In this case, C_t from Table 10.1 is 1.56 $\mu g/mL$ and k_{el} is 0.693 h^{-1}, and C_t divided by 0.693 equals 2.25 $\mu g \cdot h/mL$. Adding this value to the area from 0 to 4 h, which is 34.53, yields an area to infinite time of 36.8 $\mu g \cdot h/mL$, as in Equation 10.21.

$$\text{AUC}^{0\to4} + \text{AUC}^{4\to\infty} = \text{AUC}^{0\to\infty} = 34.53 + 2.25$$
$$= 36.8 \ \mu g \cdot h/mL \quad (10.21)$$

The area obtained from Equation 10.21 is inconsistent with the total area of 37.19 $\mu g \cdot h/mL$ in Table 10.1. Clearly, both values cannot be correct. The inconsistency between the two values lies in the 12-h data point in the table. The 12-h sample contained no detectable drug, but that does not indicate when the levels actually reached zero. It could have been reached at 9, 10, 10.5, 11, or 12 h, or any other time between 8 and 12 h postdose. The 12-h sample simply indicated that the drug level was 0 then; therefore, the triangle used to measure the small terminal area was the largest possible value. The method of end correction shows that the value was an overestimate. This overestimation may appear to be unimportant because the last portion of the AUC represents only a small fraction of the total area. However, plasma samples that are obtained during the latter period of plasma profiles are frequently separated by longer time intervals than earlier sampling times. Therefore, the terminal area may constitute a large percentage of the total area. In these cases, calculating the terminal portion of the area as accurately as possible is important.

Before leaving this topic, reviewing briefly one aspect of area values is pertinent to later discussions of bioavailability. Equation 10.16 showed that the area under the plasma curve is equal to the dose divided by the plasma clearance. Rearrangement of Equation 10.16 leads to

$$AUC^{0 \to \infty}(k_{el}) = D/V \qquad (10.22)$$

Equation 10.22 shows that the administered dose of drug, expressed as a concentration term D/V, is equal to the area under the curve multiplied by the elimination rate constant k_{el}. This relationship is important because D/V is an expression of bioavailability, or absorption efficiency. In a later chapter, similar expressions will be described for situations in which the fraction of drug absorbed is unknown, for example, after oral dosing. If the fraction is unknown, the expression D/V becomes FD/V, where F is the fraction of dose absorbed. Comparison of FD/V between two different oral dosages of a drug gives a measure of relative bioavailability, whereas comparison of FD/V from an oral dose to D/V from an intravenous dose of the same drug gives the absolute bioavailability, or absolute absorption efficiency from the oral dose. Whatever is being compared, the D/V or FD/V value is equal to the product of the area under the plasma curve and the elimination rate constant, not just the area under the curve.

There are two reasons for this equality. The first reason is that it is mathematically correct. The second reason is that it is intuitively correct. Whatever the quantity of drug absorbed, the area under the drug concentration versus time curve will be inversely proportional to the elimination rate constant. If the rate constant is increased, the area will decrease, and vice versa. Because the elimination rate constant has nothing to do with drug absorption or drug bioavailability, the contribution of that rate constant to the magnitude of the area should be removed by multiplying the area by the elimination rate constant.

The values of the elimination rate constant between oral and intravenous doses or between different formulations for the same drug should not differ, but they often do. Even when comparing two oral dosage forms, small differences in k_{el} could alter the area value to a sufficient extent to affect bioequivalence calculations. Normalizing for k_{el} removes this potential error.

Urinary Excretion Kinetics

In many instances, urinary excretion data may provide useful information in addition to blood or plasma data. For example, the degree of metabolism, the bioavailability of a drug following oral doses, renal clearance, and a variety of other useful parameters can be calculated from urinary excretion of drug or its metabolites. Plasma concentrations of some drugs are very low and difficult to measure. In these cases, urinary excretion data may provide the only means of examining drug pharmacokinetics. For the diuretic agents chlorothiazide and hydrochlorothiazide, urinary excretion data have been shown to be as good as, or better than, plasma data for bioavailability and bioequivalence determinations (3, 4).

The loss of drug from the body following intravenous bolus injection was described by the expression $A = A_0 e^{-k_{el}t}$ (Equation 10.6), where A_0 is the amount of drug initially. In that expression the only elimination rate constant reflecting drug loss from the body was the overall rate constant k_{el}. The rate of appearance of unchanged drug in the urine, dA_u/dt, can be obtained from the product of the quantity of drug in the body and the rate constant for urinary excretion, k_e, as in Equation 10.23.

$$dA_u/dt = k_e A \tag{10.23}$$

The value A is not a constant in this expression but is a constantly changing value; therefore, Equation 10.23 can be rewritten as

$$dA_u/dt = k_e A_0 e^{-k_{el}t} \tag{10.24}$$

Integration of Equation 10.24 yields

$$A_u = (k_e A_0/k_{el}) (1 - e^{-k_{el}t}) \tag{10.25}$$

This equation describes the accumulation of unchanged drug in urine with respect to time. Consider the limits of this expression when $t = 0$ and when $t = \infty$. When $t = 0$, that is, immediately after the intravenous dose is administered, $e^{-k_{el}t}$ is equal to unity because any number to the power of zero equals unity, and the parenthetical term in Equation 10.25 becomes 0, as does A_u. If t is allowed to increase to an infinitely large value, that is, a sufficiently long time for the urinary excretion of unchanged drug to be completed, then the expression $e^{-k_{el}t}$ becomes $e^{-k_{el}\infty}$, which equals zero, and A_u then becomes equal to $A_0 k_e/k_{el}$, as in

$$A_u^\infty = A_0 k_e/k_{el} \qquad (10.26)$$

Equation 10.26 can then be substituted into Equation 10.25 to obtain a new expression

$$A_u = A_u^\infty (1 - e^{-k_{el}t}) \qquad (10.27)$$

Equations 10.25 and 10.27 thus describe the continuous cumulative excretion of unchanged drug in urine, as in Figure 10.3. Note two interesting characteristics about these equations. First, the total urinary recovery of unchanged drug is equal to the dose, A_0, multiplied by the quotient k_e/k_{el}. Clearly, if k_e is equal to k_{el}, i.e., the drug is removed from the body solely by urinary excretion, then $k_e/k_{el} = 1$ and $A_u = A_0$. Thus, the quantity of drug recovered in urine is controlled by the dose and by the ratio k_e/k_{el}.

The second characteristic is that, whereas the rate constant for urinary excretion is k_e, the time course of urinary recovery, as described by Equations 10.25 and 10.27, is the overall rate constant, k_{el}. The value of k_e plays its part in the constant term in Equation 10.28 and thus determines the proportion of drug that is recovered unchanged in urine.

A great deal of information can be obtained from urinary excretion data. If sufficient collection points are taken, similar types of information can be obtained to that from plasma data, with the exception of the drug distribution volume. This parameter cannot be estimated from urinary excretion data alone because the calculations are restricted to the quantity of drug voided in urine.

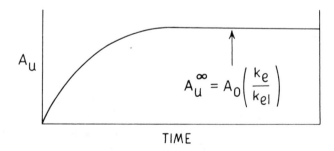

TIME

Figure 10.3. Cumulative urinary recovery of unchanged drug following rapid intravenous injection.

Construction of Sigma-Minus Plots

One very useful method of analyzing urine data is the construction of sigma-minus plots (5). This method, as the name implies, is based on the relationship between the total quantity of drug eliminated in urine minus the quantity that has been eliminated up to a certain time. Another way of describing this plot is the quantity of drug remaining to be eliminated in urine at any time.

The equation used to construct this plot is derived directly from Equation 10.27. Rearranging this equation leads to

$$A_u^\infty - A_u = A_u^\infty e^{-k_{el}t} \tag{10.28}$$

Taking logarithms of both sides of the equation yields

$$\log (A_u^\infty - A_u) = \log A_u^\infty - (k_{el}t/2.3) \tag{10.29}$$

Thus, a plot of the logarithm of the quantity of drug remaining to be eliminated in urine, $A_u^\infty - A_u$, versus time will yield a straight line with a slope of $-k_{el}/2.3$ and an intercept of $\log A_u^\infty$. This type of plot from urinary excretion data yields the overall elimination rate constant k_{el}, that is, the rate constant for total loss of drug from the body by all routes. It does not yield the urinary excretion rate constant, k_e. This is always the case regardless of the relative proportions of drug cleared by the urine and by other routes. The value of k_e can, of course, be obtained by multiplying k_{el} by A_u^∞/A_0, or A_u^∞/D as in

$$k_e = k_{el} (A_u^\infty/A_0) = k_{el} (A_u^\infty/D) \tag{10.30}$$

The metabolism rate constant, k_m, is then obtained, if metabolism occurs, by subtracting k_e from k_{el} as in Equation 10.31.

$$k_m = k_{el} - k_e \tag{10.31}$$

Some drugs that are frequently given by intravenous bolus injection, and also their biological half-lives, are given in Table 10.2.

Before leaving this topic, a word of caution is appropriate. Although urinary collection data can provide useful information, in particular cumulative drug or metabolite excretion patterns or both, obtaining accurate estimates of kinetic parameters from urinary collection data is limited by the practical limits of sampling frequency and bladder holdup. One way to avoid this type of problem is to catheterize the bladder to obtain continuous urinary recovery. Bladder catheterization is not a significant

Table 10.2—Some Drugs That Are Commonly Given by Intravenous Injection and Their Biological Half-Lives

Drug	$t_{1/2}$
Aminophylline	6 h
Cafazolin	2 h
Cimetidine	1.5–2 h
Diazepam	1–2 days
Digoxin	2 days
Fluorouracil	10 min
Furosemide	20–30 min
Gentamicin	3–4 h
Lidocaine	1.5–2 h
Phenytoin	~20 h

NOTE: The half-life of phenytoin is dose-dependent because of saturable elimination.

problem in some experimental animal studies, but is less convenient in human studies. An alternative approach to achieve adequate urine flow, and hence shorter and more accurate collection intervals, is to water-load the subject. This procedure presents the disadvantage that induced diuresis may change the elimination kinetics, particularly for those compounds whose elimination may be urine flow rate dependent.

Zero-Order Drug Input and First-Order Elimination

This situation is more complex than the intravenous bolus case because it includes a time-dependent drug input or absorption component (6). An assumption intrinsic to this model is that the rate of drug absorption is zero-order, that is, the rate is a constant and is independent of drug concentration at the absorption site. Zero-order absorption commonly occurs with intravenous infusions; therefore, understanding the kinetics underlying these infusions is important. Infusions may be over a prolonged period, for example, an intravenous drip or infusion pump, where drug levels need to be sustained over prolonged time periods, or infusions may be relatively short for 15–30 min. Short infusions are frequently used for drugs such as the aminoglycoside and cephalosporin antibiotics to avoid toxicity due to the bolus effect, and to reduce pain or embolism or both at the site of administration.

Zero-order absorption kinetics has become more common because of the recent proliferation of enteral and parenteral sustained-release products, many of which are intended to release drug at a zero-order rate. Even conventional dosage forms of some compounds have been claimed to yield zero-order absorption. So, this model is important for several different types of drug dosage forms and routes of administration.

The model is depicted in Scheme 10.2. All of the symbols are identical to the intravenous bolus case except for the additional zero-order rate constant, k_0.

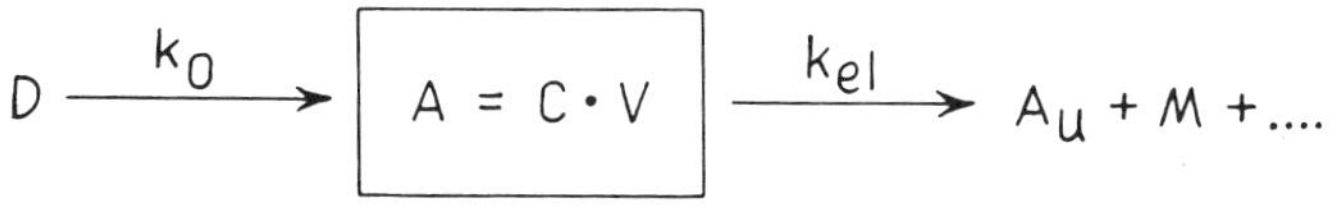

$$D \xrightarrow{\quad k_0 \quad} \boxed{A = C \cdot V} \xrightarrow{\quad k_{el} \quad} A_u + M + \ldots$$

Scheme 10.2. One-compartment open model with zero-order absorption and first-order elimination: k_0 is the zero-order rate constant for drug administration.

From the model, the rate Equation 10.32 can be written to describe the rate of change in the amount of drug in the body with respect to time.

$$dA/dt = k_0 - k_{el}A \tag{10.32}$$

In this equation, k_0 is a constant input rate that will continue as long as drug is available to be absorbed, or until the infusion is stopped. The infusion rate may be written also as D/T, where D is the dose and T is the total absorption or infusion time. Although the input rate is constant, the elimination rate is variable and obeys first-order kinetics, as in the intravenous case. The elimination rate is dependent on the product of the constant, k_{el}, and the amount of drug in the body, A.

During the initial period of zero-order input, the amount of drug in the body, A, will be small. Thus, the product $k_{el}A$ will also be small, the rate of drug input will exceed the rate of drug output, and the quantity of drug in the body will increase. As the value of A increases, the product $k_{el}A$ will also increase, so the overall rate of drug elimination will approach and eventually become equal to the rate of input. A steady state is thus achieved in which the rate of absorption equals the rate of elimination.

The infusion may be stopped either before or after the amount of drug in the body has reached steady state. During the resulting postabsorption phase, drug levels will decline at a first-order rate as in the intravenous bolus case. The two possible situations are shown in Figure 10.4.

Integration of Equation 10.32 yields Equation 10.33, which in concentration terms becomes Equation 10.34.

$$A = (k_0/k_{el}) (1 - e^{-k_{el}t}) \tag{10.33}$$

$$C = (k_0/V \cdot k_{el}) (1 - e^{-k_{el}t}) \tag{10.34}$$

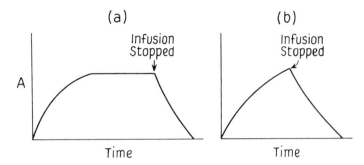

Figure 10.4. Time course of the quantity of Drug A in the body during and following zero-order infusion. In (a), the drug levels had reached steady state before the infusion was stopped, and in (b), the levels had not reached steady state.

Although two rate constants are involved in the overall drug profile, only one time-dependent function, $e^{-k_{el}t}$, is involved. If $t = 0$, $e^{-k_{el}t}$ becomes equal to unity, and $C = 0$. As the time after the start of infusion increases, the value $e^{-k_{el}t}$ becomes progressively smaller, $1 - e^{-k_{el}t}$ increases, and the accumulation curve in Figure 10.3 is obtained. If the infusion is continued for a sufficiently long period so that $e^{-k_{el}t}$ approaches or becomes zero, then the parenthetical term becomes unity, and $C = k_0/Vk_{el}$ as in

$$C_{ss} = k_0/Vk_{el} \qquad (10.35)$$

Because the steady-state concentration is described, C is now expressed as C_{ss}.

Thus, at steady state, as in Figure 10.4a, the concentration of drug in the distribution volume is equal to the infusion rate, k_0, divided by the plasma clearance, Vk_{el}. Because the constant k_0 has units of mass per unit time, and because plasma clearance is commonly expressed in terms of volume per unit time, C_{ss} has units of mass per volume, or concentration.

The relationship in Equation 10.35 provides a considerable amount of information. For example, knowledge of plasma clearance and drug infusion rate permits calculation of the steady-state drug concentration in plasma. Alternatively, if k_0 and C_{ss} are known, then the plasma clearance can be calculated. Similarly, if k_0, C_{ss}, and the elimination $t_{1/2}$ are known, then the distribution volume can be calculated.

If both sides of Equation 10.35 are multiplied by the distribution volume, V, Equation 10.36 is obtained.

$$A_{ss} = k_0/k_{el} \qquad (10.36)$$

This equation describes the amount of drug in the body at steady state (A_{ss}) in terms of the absorption and elimination rate constants. Thus, the total body drug load can be determined by dividing the zero-order infusion rate constant by the first-order elimination rate constant. Thus, A_{ss} can be determined without knowing C_{ss}.

As previously noted from Equations 10.34 and 10.35, steady-state drug levels are dependent on both the infusion and elimination rate constants. Faster infusion yields higher blood levels; faster elimination yields lower blood levels. However, from Equation 10.34, the time dependency of the accumulation process is clearly dependent only on the elimination rate constant k_{el}. No matter how fast a drug is infused, the time to reach steady state is governed exclusively by the elimination rate constant. How long it will take for a drug level to reach steady state can be determined from Equation 10.34. Because this equation is exponential, steady state will theoretically take a very long time to achieve. But because pharmacokineticists have to consider practicalities, 95% of steady state may be considered a reasonable approximation, given the normal variability of biological data. How long does a drug need to be infused before drug levels in the blood reach 95% of the steady-state values? To calculate this, Equation 10.34 can be rewritten in the form of Equation 10.37.

$$95 = 100 (1 - e^{-k_{el}t}) \tag{10.37}$$

From this equation, and from the relationship that $0.693/k_{el} = t_{1/2}$, t becomes equal to $4.3\ t_{1/2}$. Thus, whatever the infusion rate, 4.3 (or approximately 4.5) drug elimination half-lives will be needed to reach 95% of steady state values. Consider some examples. If a drug has a biological half-life of 1 h, then the drug would need to be infused for about 4.5 h before steady-state levels were approached. If the infusion rate were doubled, steady-state levels would also be doubled, but the new levels would not be reached any faster. If on the other hand, the drug half-life was 24 h, 4.5 days would be needed to approach steady state.

Regardless of the infusion rate, the time required to reach steady state, or the time period during which circulating drug levels are below or have not yet approached those levels required for therapeutic efficacy, cannot be reduced provided k_{el} remains constant. This situation occurs not only with drugs that have long biological half-lives, but also with drugs whose elimination half-lives are normally short but may be prolonged in disease conditions such as renal failure.

An appreciation of the need to understand the important relationships in Equations 10.34 and 10.37 can be obtained by considering the cardiac glycoside digoxin. This drug frequently has to be administered by infusion. If a patient received an intravenous infusion of digoxin, and a digoxin blood concentration was determined 2 h after the start of infusion, could the drug concentration at that time be assumed to be at steady state? Digoxin has a biological half-life of approximately 2 days so that the time required for blood levels to reach steady state during a continuous infusion is 9 days. After 2 h of infusion, the digoxin concentration can be calculated from Equation 10.34 by setting k_{el} equal to 0.693/48, or 0.014 h^{-1}, t equal to 2 h, and k_0/Vk_{el} equal to 1, or 100%. Substituting these numerical values into Equation 10.34, as in Equation 10.38, yields a concentration value at 2 h that is only 2.8% of the steady-state value.

$$C - 100 (1 - e^{-0.014 \times 2}) = 2.8\% \qquad (10.38)$$

If the assumption had been made that steady state had been achieved at 2 h into the infusion, and drug levels at that time were within the therapeutic range, then continued infusion beyond 2 h would undoubtedly have produced toxic drug concentrations.

In cases of prolonged drug accumulation, a bolus loading dose often has to be administered to achieve required therapeutic levels at an early time. Under most circumstances, a convenient approach is to administer a loading dose that will instantaneously achieve the drug concentration, or total body load, that gives the desired therapeutic response at steady state. This situation is achieved by administering a bolus dose equal to k_0/k_{el}. Because k_0 has units of mass per unit time and because k_{el} has units of reciprocal time, the quotient has units of mass.

Consider the time course of events if a bolus dose of magnitude k_0/k_{el} is administered as a bolus injection and at the same time an infusion is started at a zero-order rate k_0. The resulting time course of the quantity of drug in the body is given by

$$A = k_0/k_{el} \, e^{-k_{el}t} + k_0/k_{el} (1 - e^{-k_{el}t}) \qquad (10.39)$$

The two components to Equation 10.39 are a decreasing component that results from the elimination of the bolus dose, and an increasing component that results from the infusion.

Equation 10.39 can be substantially simplified to

$$A = k_0/k_{el} \qquad (10.40)$$

This equation indicates that the quantity of drug in the body is constant from the time that the bolus-loading dose is administered until the end of the infusion. This elegant relationship is due to control of both the decline in drug levels following the loading dose and the increase in drug levels from the infusion by the elimination rate constant k_{el}. Therefore, the decreasing and increasing drug profiles are mirror images of each other, and the sum of the quantites of drug in the body from the loading and infusion doses will always equal k_0/k_{el}, as shown in Figure 10.5.

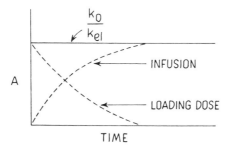

Figure 10.5. Quantity of drug in the body following a loading intravenous bolus dose, k_0/k_{el}, and a zero-order infusion initiated at the same time as the bolus injection.

This example is, of course, the simplest. For very potent drugs, dividing the loading dose into two smaller doses to approach steady state in a stepwise, cautious fashion is more appropriate. Two smaller doses will reduce the initial drug levels, but will essentially achieve the same goal of rapidly attaining steady-state levels while minimizing toxic effects.

Oral doses are more complicated because the bolus dose will probably be absorbed by a first-order process rather than be instantaneously available in the circulation. However, provided the absorption rate is fast compared to the elimination rate, the concepts embodied in Equation 10.39 still apply.

What happens to drug levels when the infusion, or any zero-order drug absorption process, stops? Consider Figure 10.4 and Equations 10.34 and 10.35. Assume the situation in Figure 10.4a, that is, steady-state drug levels are achieved during infusion. In this case, the declining drug levels obtained after the infusion has stopped will be described by Equation 10.41.

$$C = k_0/Vk_{el}\, e^{-k_{el}t'} \qquad (10.41)$$

where t' is the time elapsed since the end of the infusion. The drug profile at the end of the infusion is essentially identical to that after an intravenous bolus dose except that C_0 or D/V from the intravenous bolus dose case is replaced by k_0/Vk_{el}.

Assume now the situation in Figure 10.4b. In this case, steady state

Table 10.3—Some Drugs That Are Commonly Given by Intravenous Infusion and Their Biological Half-Lives

Drug	$t_{1/2}$
Aminophylline	6 h
Amphotericin	1–2 days
Cyclophosphamide	3–6 h
Digoxin	2 days
Gentamicin	3–4 h
Heparin	1–2 h
Lidocaine	1.5–2 h
Nitroglycerin	~30 min
Verapamil	3–6 h

has not been achieved before zero-order infusion is stopped; therefore, at that time the drug level is given by Equation 10.42.

$$C = k_0/Vk_{el} (1 - e^{-k_{el}T}) \qquad (10.42)$$

where T is the total zero-order infusion time. The postabsorptive drug concentrations in this situation are described by

$$C = k_0/Vk_{el} (1 - e^{-k_{el}T}) e^{-k_{el}t'} \qquad (10.43)$$

where t' has the same meaning as in Equation 10.41. This situation is again identical to that following an intravenous bolus dose except that C_0 from the intravenous case is replaced by the more complex term in Equation 10.43.

The situation described by Equation 10.43 is common for orally administered dosage forms that are designed to release drug in zero-order fashion. The most suitable drug candidates for sustained release, as discussed earlier, have elimination half-lives between 2 and 8 h. For those drugs with the shortest half-life in this range, 4.5 half-lives, or 9 h, would be needed to approach steady-state levels in the body. On the other hand, drugs with a half-life of 8 h would take 36 h to approach steady-state values. As far as drug absorption is concerned, the residence time in the GI tract may be considered to be approximately 12 h (as mentioned earlier, there is much disagreement on this value). Therefore, only those drugs that have short half-lives of approximately 2 h will achieve steady-state blood levels from a single oral dose, and postabsorption blood profiles can be described by Equation 10.41. Drugs with elimination half-lives longer than 2 h will not achieve steady-state levels after a single oral dose, and their postabsorptive blood profiles are likely to be described by Equation 10.43. The problem of GI transit time, and its limiting influence on the available time for release of orally administered drugs, has led to a number of formulations designed specifically, with variable degrees of success, to remain in the GI tract for longer periods and so allow more time for drug release. Some drugs that are frequently given by zero-order intravenous infusion are listed in Table 10.3.

Summary

1. Following bolus intravenous injection of a drug that obeys one-compartment model kinetics, plasma profiles can be used to estimate the elimination rate constant, half-life, apparent distribution volume, and plasma clearance.

2. Urinary excretion data can be utilized to calculate renal clearance.

3. Areas under drug profiles in plasma can be determined analytically, or measured by the trapezoidal rule or log trapezoidal rule. The area under the curve, normalized by elimination rate constant where appropriate, provides a measure of drug absorption efficiency.

4. For an intravenously administered drug, sigma-minus plots of urinary excretion data can be used to calculate rate constants for drug excretion and metabolism.

5. Zero-order drug absorption may occur, not only with intravenous infusions, but also with a variety of sustained-release dosage forms.

6. Drug concentrations in plasma during zero-order administration are controlled by the rates of administration and elimination. The time to reach steady-state drug levels is controlled only by the elimination rate constant.

7. Bolus loading dose for an infused drug can be calculated from the ratio of infusion and elimination rate constants.

Literature Cited

1. Shargel, L.; Yu, A. B. C. *Applied Biopharmaceutics and Pharmacokinetics*; Appleton-Century-Crofts: New York, 1980; pp 28–37.
2. Wagner, J. G.; Northam, J. I. *J. Pharm. Sci.*, **1967**, 56, 529–531.
3. Osman, M. A.; Patel, R. B.; Irwin, D. S.; Craig, W. A.; Welling, P. G. *Biopharm. Drug Dispos.* **1982**, 3, 89–94.
4. Barbhaiya, R. H.; Craig, W. A.; Corrick-West, H. P.; Welling, P. G. *J. Pharm. Sci.*, **1982**, 71, 245–248.
5. Wagner, J. G. *Fundamentals of Clinical Pharmacokinetics*; Drug Intelligence Publications: Hamilton, IL, 1975; pp 77–78.
6. Rodriguez, N.; Madsen, P. O.; Welling, P. G. *Antimicrob. Ag. Chemother.*, **1979**, 15, 465–469.

Problems

1. Equal quantities of two different drugs are administered to a patient by rapid intravenous (IV) injection. Neither drug binds to proteins. The concentration of Drug A in plasma immediately after dosing is 10 µg/mL, and the concentration of Drug B is 20 µg/mL. Drug A has a biological half-life double that of Drug B. Which drug has the greater plasma clearance?

2. Following a 250-mg intravenous bolus dose of a drug, the resulting drug concentrations in plasma declined in an apparent monoexponential manner. Extrapolation of the log-linear elimination slope to time zero yielded a concentration of 12.5 µg/mL. At 2 h after dosing, the concentration had declined to 6.25 µg/mL. What is the plasma clearance of the drug?

3. If the drug in problem 2 is cleared from the body 25% via the kidneys and 75% via hepatic metabolism, what will be the ratio of its renal clearance to plasma clearance?

4. One hour after a bolus IV injection of 100 mg of a drug that has a biological half-life of 4 h, the concentration of unchanged drug in serum was 1.7 µg/mL. What is the apparent distribution volume of the drug?

5. A 200-mg dose of a drug is injected intravenously into a human subject. The drug rapidly distributes into an apparently homogeneous fluid volume. Ten hours after injection, the plasma concentration of drug is 3.28 µg/mL. At 16.92 hours after injection the plasma concentration of drug is 1.64 µg/mL. Calculate (i) the biological half-life, (ii) elimination rate constant, (iii) volume of distribution, and (iv) plasma clearance.

6. Following IV bolus injection, the following drug plasma concentrations were obtained:

Time (h)	Concentration (µg/mL)
0	100
0.5	77.9
1	60.7
2	36.8
3	22.3
4	13.5

Calculate (i) the trapezoidal area under the plasma curve from $t = 0$ to $t = 4$ h, and (ii) the area from zero to infinite time.

7. After an intravenous bolus injection of 250 mg of a drug, which distributes into a single homogeneous volume of 12 L in the body and is cleared completely as unchanged drug in urine, the following urinary excretion data were obtained:

Time After Dosing (h)	Cumulative Urinary Recovery of Drug (mg)
0.5	16.9
1.0	32.7
2.0	61.1
4.0	107.2
8.0	168.5
12.0	203.4
24.0	241.3
48.0	249.7
96.0	250.0

Calculate the following:
  (i) By sigma-minus plot, the drug elimination half-life.
 (ii) Plasma clearance.
(iii) Renal clearance.
 (iv) The concentration of drug in plasma immediately after and at 1 h after dosing.
  (v) The area under the drug plasma curve from zero to infinite time.

8. A drug is administered to a 70-kg male patient by means of a constant rate IV infusion at 0.5 mg/min. The drug has a biological half-life of 4.5 h and appears to distribute into a space equivalent to that of blood volume (5 L). Calculate the following:
  (i) The steady-state plasma level achieved with the infusion.
 (ii) The time taken to reach 95% and 99% of the steady-state levels.

9. Another 70-kg male patient receives the same infusion as in problem 8. However, this patient has also been taking another drug that has induced his drug metabolizing enzymes. This drug causes the half-life of the infused drug to be reduced to 1.5 h. Recalculate the following:
  (i) The steady-state plasma levels achieved in this case.
 (ii) The time taken to reach 95% and 99% of the steady-state levels.

10. The steady-state levels obtained in problem 9 are now too low for therapeutic efficacy. What would the constant rate infusion have to be adjusted to in order to achieve the steady-state levels of drug in problem 8? Does altering the infusion rate in this way influence the time required to reach the steady state?

11. From the data in problem 10, calculate the drug plasma concentration at 1 h and 10 h after the infusion has stopped.

12. For the situation described in problem 8, how much drug would have to be given as an initial bolus injection to achieve the required steady-state plasma level instantaneously?

11

The One-Compartment Open Model with First-Order Absorption and Elimination

When drugs are taken orally, or by intramuscular or subcutaneous injection, the resulting drug profile in plasma can frequently be described by a pharmacokinetic model that incorporates first-order absorption and elimination. First-order absorption and elimination occurs, or appears to occur, in the great majority of cases after oral dosing, regardless of whether the dose is given as a solution, suspension, capsule, tablet, or controlled-release product.

General Aspects of First-Order Absorption and Elimination

Interpretation of the absorption phase of such drug profiles in terms of a first-order rate constant is intuitive when drug is given as a solution. One might expect that the rate of absorption would be dependent upon the mucosal:serosal concentration gradient generated by the solution dose. But the absorption process for solid oral dosage forms is more complex and may be influenced by the dissolution rate of solid products, stomach emptying, and a variety of other factors. It is surprising that, in most instances, the first-order approach is a reasonable approximation to the overall absorption process and often gives a good description of the data. Other absorption models have been proposed for particular drugs and formulations. However, these models are frequently difficult

0065–7719/86/0185–0163$07.00/1
© 1986 American Chemical Society

to prove, and the first-order absorption model still appears to provide the most generally used description of the absorption phase.

The model is shown in Scheme 11.1. This model has two major differences from the models for intravenous administration. The first difference is the introduction of a first-order absorption constant, k_a, so that the rate of absorption becomes dose dependent. The second difference is the additional parameter, F, which describes the absorption efficiency, or the fraction of the dose, D, that is absorbed into the systemic circulation.

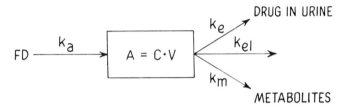

Scheme 11.1. One-compartment open model with first-order elimination, where F is the fraction of the dose, D, absorbed from the dosage site into the systemic circulation, and k_a is the first-order rate constant for drug absorption.

After intravenous injection, the parameter F was not pertinent because the availability of administered drug is almost always 100%; therefore, F was equal to unity. However, after oral doses, and also after intramuscular doses in some cases, bioavailability is not always 100%. Complete absorption from oral doses tends to be the exception rather than the rule. Incomplete absorption might be expected because of the phenomena occurring in the GI tract. After intramuscular doses, more efficient absorption might be expected, but this is not always the case. Incomplete absorption from intramuscular doses is due in part to degradation of drug at the intramuscular site, drug precipitation, or very slow release of a portion of the drug that leads to low and perhaps undetectable drug levels during prolonged periods. Intramuscularly dosed phenobarbital has been shown to be only 80% bioavailable compared to oral doses in humans (1), and intramuscularly dosed promethazine has been shown to be approximately 70-80% bioavailable in dogs compared to intravenously dosed drug (2). The possibility of first-order degradation of drug at the absorption site, whether gastrointestinal or intramuscular, introduces another complicating factor that affects the magnitude and interpretation of k_a.

Suppose that a drug is at the absorption site and is simultaneously being absorbed at a rate governed by an intrinsic absorption rate constant

k_{ab}. Also, suppose the drug is enzymatically degraded at a rate governed by a rate constant k_d. The overall rate of drug loss from the absorption site is then governed by the sum of k_{ab} and k_d. Because k_a is used to describe the overall loss of drug from the absorption site, the amount of drug X remaining at the absorption site at any time is described by

$$X = FDe^{-(k_{ab}+k_d)t} = FDe^{-k_a t} \tag{11.1}$$

Previously, the apparent rate constant for appearance of intravenously dosed drug in the urine was shown to be equal to the overall elimination rate constant, k_{el}. Similarly, the apparent rate constant for appearance of orally or intramuscularly dosed drug into the circulation is equal to the overall rate constant for loss of drug from that absorption site by all processes. In other words, the rate constant that is obtained from the drug concentration curve in plasma is not necessarily the intrinsic absorption rate constant but may be a constant related to overall loss of drug from the absorption site. An observed k_a may actually be the sum of k_{ab}, k_d, and any other rate constant that contributes to loss of drug from the absorption site.

   An interesting analogy can be drawn with ocular drug administration (3). When a drug solution is applied to the surface of the eye, for example from an eye dropper, more than 95% of the drug is washed from the eye surface by tear movement and is washed down the nasolachrymal duct. Thus, the overall rate of loss of drug from the absorption site at the surface of the eye is very fast. Absorption of drug into the eye will continue only as long as drug is available at the absorption site. Because the overall loss of drug from the eye surface is approximately a first-order process, the apparent rate constant for drug penetration into the eye is very fast, and the absorption rate constant calculated from drug levels within the eye may overestimate the actual intrinsic absorption rate constant by a factor of 20 or more. This concept is worth remembering when considering drug absorption kinetics. From Scheme 11.1, Equation 11.2 can be written to describe the rate of change in the amount of drug, A, in the body.

$$dA/dt = k_a X - k_{el} A \tag{11.2}$$

In this equation, X is the amount of drug remaining to be absorbed as described in Equation 11.1. By substituting for X from Equation 11.1 and then integrating, Equation 11.3 is obtained.

$$A = FD\,[k_a/(k_a - k_{el})]\,(e^{-k_{el}t} - e^{-k_a t}) \tag{11.3}$$

This equation can then be converted to describe time-dependent drug concentrations by dividing both sides by the distribution volume, V, to

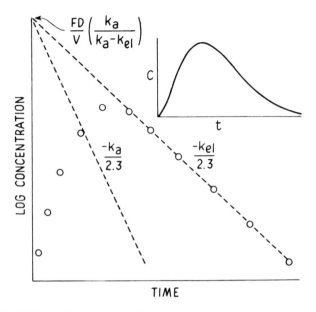

Figure 11.1. Plot of the logarithm of drug concentration versus time for a drug that obeys one-compartment model kinetics with first-order absorption and elimination. The concentration is plotted on a linear scale in the inset.

obtain Equation 11.4, which describes the drug profile that is shown in Figure 11.1.

$$C = FD/V \, [k_a/(k_a - k_{el})] \, (e^{-k_{el}t} - e^{-k_a t}) \qquad (11.4)$$

Because the kinetic parameters associated with the one-compartment model with first-order absorption and elimination have been identified, the next step is to understand how numerical values are assigned to the parameters from a drug concentration profile. Understanding the variable relationship among k_a, the absorption rate constant, and k_{el}, the elimination rate constant, is important. Three different situations can occur as follows:

1. k_a may be greater than k_{el}.

2. k_a may be less than k_{el}.

3. The two constants may have the same, or approximately the same, numerical value.

In most instances, the first case occurs. The absorption rate constant (or the apparent absorption rate constant) of a drug is usually greater than the elimination rate constant. However, for drugs that have short biological half-lives of perhaps 1 h or less, and also for drugs that are absorbed slowly, the elimination rate constant may be greater than the absorption rate constant. Also, in many cases the values of the two constants may be so similar that they become indistinguishable.

Graphical Estimation of Some Kinetic Parameters

Case 1. In the most usual case, k_a is greater than k_{el}. Equation 11.4 shows that both of the exponential terms equal unity at time zero; C is therefore equal to 0. As time increases after dosing, the values of the exponential terms gradually diminish from unity toward zero, but the exponential term containing k_a (in this case, the larger rate constant) will approach zero at a faster rate than the term containing k_{el}. Therefore, after a certain time, the exponential term containing k_a becomes so small that Equation 11.4 reduces to

$$C - FD/V \ [k_a/(k_a - k_{el})] \ e^{-k_{el}t} \tag{11.5}$$

This equation, in logarithmic form, becomes

$$\log C = \log \{FD/V \ [k_a/(k_a - k_{el})]\} - (k_{el}/2.3)t \tag{11.6}$$

Equation 11.6 describes a linear relationship between the logarithm of C and time, which has a slope of $-k_{el}/2.3$ and an intercept of $FD/V[k_a/(k_a - k_{el})]$. This linear postabsorptive phase is shown in Figure 11.1.

A suitable method to obtain k_a is the method of curve stripping, or residuals. If Equation 11.4 is subtracted from Equation 11.5, the residual Equation 11.7 is obtained, which can be written in logarithmic form as Equation 11.8.

$$R = FD/V \ [k_a/(k_a - k_{el})] \ e^{-k_a t} \tag{11.7}$$

$$\log R = \log \{FD/V \ [k_a/(k_a - k_{el})]\} - k_a/2.3 \ t \tag{11.8}$$

Equation 11.8 is identical to Equation 11.6 except that the slope is a function of k_a instead of k_{el}. Equation 11.8 was obtained by subtracting the equation describing the entire drug profile from the equation describing the extrapolated terminal phase. Equation 11.8 can also be obtained graphically as shown in Figure 11.1 by subtracting the actual data points during the absorptive phase from the values on the extrapolated elimination slope. If these residuals are plotted against time, an estimate of k_a is obtained. The intercepts of the terminal slope, from Equation 11.6, and the residual slope, from Equation 11.8, at time zero are identical. If they

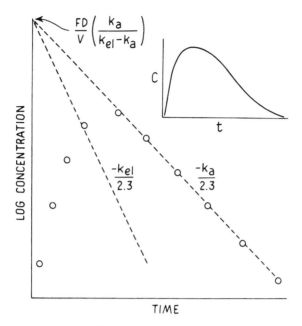

Figure 11.2. Interpretation of log C versus time profile for a drug that obeys one-compartment model kinetics and for which the first-order absorption rate constant, k_a, is smaller than the first-order elimination rate constant, k_{el}.

were not identical in practice, or nearly identical given usual biological data noise, then the model may be incorrect; nonlinear kinetics may be operative, or an absorption lag time may exist. Both of these situations will be discussed later.

From the curve-stripping procedures, estimates of k_a, k_{el}, and their associated half-lives have been obtained. The numerical value of the common intercept from both the terminal and residual slopes is also known. Therefore, the values of k_a and k_{el} can be substituted into the measured intercept value to solve for FD/V. The drug-concentration profile has been described mathematically in terms of the model using two rate constants and a concentration term, FD/V, which describes the overall drug absorption efficiency.

To further resolve the function FD/V, solving for F, the fraction of dose absorbed, or V, the drug distribution volume in the body, is necessary. However, neither of these parameters can be solved unless additional data, such as urinary excretion or intravenous data, are available. If the quantity of drug absorbed, F, is known by comparison with intravenous data, then V can be calculated. On the other hand, if V is known, then the value F can be calculated. However, in the absence of such data, the function FD/V cannot be further resolved. But even if unresolved, form FD/V is a useful parameter, as demonstrated later in this chapter.

Case 2. In the second kind of relationship between absorption and elimination rate constants, k_a is less than k_{el}. The equation that describes the drug concentration profile in this case is identical to the first case because the form of the equation is independent of the numerical values of the constants. However, the numerical values do influence how the equation is used to analyze the data.

Equation 11.4 is again appropriate for the analysis. However, in this case, k_a is less than k_{el}, so both of the parenthetical terms in the equation become negative. Equation 11.4 rearranges to Equation 11.9, in which both parenthetical terms become positive.

$$C = FD/V \ [k_a/(k_{el} - k_a)] \ (e^{-k_a t} - e^{-k_{el} t}) \tag{11.9}$$

Because k_{el} is greater than k_a, the product $k_{el}t$ will increase with increasing time values at a faster rate than the product $k_a t$ so that the exponential term $e^{-k_{el} t}$ will be the first of the two exponential terms to approach zero and drop out of the equation. At that time, Equation 11.9 reduces to Equation 11.10, which can be written in logarithmic form as Equation 11.11.

$$C = FD/V \ [k_a/(k_{el} - k_a)] \ e^{-k_a t} \tag{11.10}$$

$$\log C = \log \{FD/V \ [(k_a/(k_{el} - k_a)]\} - (k_a/2.3) \ t \tag{11.11}$$

Thus, the terminal declining phase of the drug-level curve, which in the first example was controlled by the elimination rate constant, k_{el}, is now controlled by the absorption rate constant k_a.

If residuals are taken between Equations 11.10 and 11.9 in analogous fashion to that described previously between Equations 11.4 and 11.5, the residual is described by Equation 11.12, which in logarithmic form becomes Equation 11.13.

$$R = FD/V \ [k_a/(k_{el} - k_a)] \ e^{-k_{el} t} \tag{11.12}$$

$$\log R = \log \{FD/V \ [k_a/(k_{el} - k_a)]\} - (k_{el}/2.3) \ t \tag{11.13}$$

Thus, the residual slope gives the elimination rate constant k_{el}. Also, the common intercept of the terminal and the residual lines at the y intercept at time zero differs from the analogous intercept when k_a was greater than k_{el} because the values of k_a and k_{el} are transposed in the denominator.

This model, in which k_a is less than k_{el}, has been called the "flip-flop" model, for obvious reasons. Failure to recognize the possibility of this model may cause gross misinterpretation of data. This model is not rare, and may apply to drugs that have short biological half-lives, drugs that exhibit prolonged absorption, and combinations of these.

The situation just described leads to the question of which model is correct. How can the larger of the two rate constants, k_a or k_{el}, be determined? Sometimes assigning the correct values is straightforward. For example, with drugs like digoxin or phenobarbital, which have biological half-lives of 2 and 4 days, respectively, and even with drugs like tetracycline, which has a half-life of 8 to 10 h, it is intuitively obvious which of the rate constants is k_a and which is k_{el}. Because of the limited residence time the drug has in which to be absorbed from the GI tract, drug levels cannot possibly be prolonged over many hours or days in the situation where k_a is small relative to k_{el}, at least with GI absorption. Absorption would stop when drug was voided from the GI tract, the absorption phase would be truncated, and a much less prolonged profile than that actually observed would result. However, for drugs that have relatively short elimination half-lives of less than 4-6 h, correctly identifying the absorption and elimination rate constants may be difficult. The method of analyzing data with this model is summarized in Figure 11.2, which is analogous to Figure 11.1.

Case 3. In the third kind of relationship between absorption and elimination rate constants, k_a is equal to k_{el}. Theoretically the two values will never be the same. However, the values may often be very similar, and with the normal biological and individual variations that regularly occur in pharmacokinetics, the values can frequently become indistinguishable. The methods used for the first two situations cannot be used in this case. If k_a is set equal to k_{el} in Equation 11.4 or in Equation 11.9, then both equations become equal to zero. The correct rate equation for this model is Equation 11.14, where k is the common value of the absorption and elimination rate constants.

$$dA/dt = kX - kA = k(X - A) \tag{11.14}$$

If X is defined as in Equation 11.1, Equation 11.14 becomes

$$dA/dt = k\,(FDe^{-kt} - A) \tag{11.15}$$

Integrating this expression and converting to concentration terms yields

$$C = FDkte^{-kt}/V \tag{11.16}$$

This equation is quite different from Equations 11.9 and 11.14. The coefficient now contains the value of time, and is therefore no longer a constant. Thus, although there is only one exponential term, which normally yields a straight line when plotted against time on semilogarithmic graph paper, a straight line cannot be obtained during any phase of the drug-level profile, be it absorption or elimination. Instead, a continuous convex curve is obtained. This situation frequently occurs. In practice, locating a linear elimination phase in a drug profile is frequently difficult. Maybe the linear elimination phase is not there! A true terminal linear phase may not exist, but probably the curve is completely curvilinear because of the similarity or identity of the absorption and elimination rate constants.

Other Parameters Associated with First-Order Absorption and Elimination

Further examination of the two cases where k_a does not equal k_{el} is necessary because these cases are the most common. Apart from the constants that have already been extracted from the data, such as k_a, k_{el}, their associated half-lives, and FD/V, several other useful parameters can be derived. Three parameters that are frequently used, particularly in bioavailability or bioequivalence studies, are the maximum drug concentration in plasma, C_{max}, the time of the maximum drug concentration, T_{max}, and the area under the drug concentration profile $AUC^{0 \to t}$ or $AUC^{0 \to \infty}$. Together, C_{max}, T_{max}, and AUC provide an almost complete description of a drug concentration profile.

The maximum drug concentration in the bloodstream, C_{max}, occurs at time T_{max}, which is the time when the drug profile is at its peak and the slope of the drug profile is changing sign, that is, the first derivative of Equation 11.4 and Equation 11.9 equals zero, as in Equation 11.17.

$$FD/V[k_a/(k_a - k_{el})](-k_{el}e^{-k_{el}T_{max}} + k_a e^{-k_a T_{max}}) = 0 \qquad (11.17)$$

The first part of this equation, $FD/V[k_a/(k_a - k_{el})]$, cannot equal zero because it comprises a constant. If this constant were zero, then the drug level would be zero at all values of t. Therefore, the exponential terms in parentheses must equal zero, as in

$$k_{el}e^{-k_{el}T_{max}} = k_a e^{-k_a T_{max}} \qquad (11.18)$$

By simple rearrangement and taking logarithms, this expression can be written as

$$T_{max} = [1/(k_a - k_{el})] \ln (k_a/k_{el}) \qquad (11.19)$$

This equation shows that T_{max} is a function of the relative magnitude of the absorption and elimination rate constants k_a and k_{el}. The data in Table 11.1 show that the value of T_{max} is inversely related to both rate constants; T_{max} is delayed when the absorption rate is decreased, and also when the elimination rate is decreased, but not to quite the same extent. A fourfold alteration in the value of k_a causes a 2.5-fold alteration in the value of T_{max}. On the other hand, a tenfold alteration in k_{el} is required to have a similar effect on the value of T_{max}.

Table 11.1—Influence of k_a and k_{el} on T_{max}

$k_a(h^{-1})$	$k_{el}(h^{-1})$	$C_{max}(h)$
2.0	0.1	1.6
1.0	0.1	2.6
0.5	0.1	4.0
1.0	0.5	1.4
1.0	0.1	2.6
1.0	0.05	3.2

NOTE: Data were generated from Equation 11.19.

The value of C_{max} can be determined in a similar fashion to that for T_{max} and is given by

$$C_{max} = (FD/V) \, (k_a/k_{el})^{k_{el}/(k_{el} - k_a)} \tag{11.20}$$

This expression is different in many ways from Equation 11.19 for T_{max}, but the primary difference is that the concentration term FD/V, in addition to the rate constants, is included. In other words, C_{max} is drug concentration-dependent and absorption efficiency-dependent, whereas T_{max} is not. The data in Table 11.2 show that, whereas the value of T_{max} is inversely related to the absorption and elimination rate constants, the

Table 11.2—Influence of k_a and k_{el} on C_{max}

$k_a(h^{-1})$	$k_{el}(h^{-1})$	$T_{max}(h)$
2.0	0.1	0.68
1.0	0.1	0.46
0.5	0.1	0.21
1.0	0.5	0.01
1.0	0.1	0.46
1.0	0.05	0.67

NOTE: Data were generated from Equation 11.20, and FD/V was assumed to equal 100 µg/mL.

value of C_{max} is positively related to k_a but inversely related to k_{el}. This relationship makes good intuitive sense. A slower absorption rate constant produces a flatter drug profile and a lower value for C_{max}. A slower elimination rate constant, on the other hand, permits blood levels to increase to a greater extent during the absorption phase, and a higher C_{max} value results.

Drug Absorption Plots

Searching for a satisfactory manner to describe drug absorption as a function of time, Wagner and Nelson developed a method that applies only to the one-compartment model (4). For the two-compartment model, the alternative Loo–Riegelman method should be used (5). Because the Loo–Riegelman method is simply a modification of the one-compartment model approach, attention will focus here on the Wagner–Nelson method. To repeat the Wagner–Nelson derivation here would not be useful. The derivation is elegantly simple, based on mass balance principles, and culminates in Equation 11.21.

$$\text{percent absorbed} = \frac{C_t + k_{el} \int_0^t C \, dt \times 100}{k_{el} \int_0^\infty C \, dt} \tag{11.21}$$

The numerator of this equation is the sum of the drug concentration at time t and the product of the drug elimination rate constant and the area under the drug concentration curve from zero to time t. The denominator is the elimination rate constant multiplied by the area from zero to infinite time. The denominator is thus the limiting value for the numerator. That is, when C_t has dropped to zero, the drug concentration profile is concluded, and all drug that is going to be absorbed will have been absorbed. Thus, after all drug is absorbed, Equation 11.21 must equal unity, or 100%.

The example in Table 11.3 demonstrates how the Wagner–Nelson-method is used. As shown in the table, the Wagner–Nelson method consists of listing the drug concentration in plasma at each sampling time; calculating the cumulative area under the blood curve up to that time; multiplying each area by the elimination rate constant k_{el}, which is obtained from the terminal log-linear portion of the curve; and adding the drug concentration in plasma at the particular sampling time. Thus, a series of gradually increasing values is obtained. In this example, an average maximum value of 9.407 is obtained. Each of the preceding values is then expressed as a percentage of the maximum. The cumulative per-

centages of the drug that is going to eventually be absorbed is represented
at each time point. In this case, the drug is 69.7% absorbed at 3 h, 86%
at 8 h, and 100% at 15 h. A plot of the percentage absorbed versus time
provides a useful picture of how rapidly absorption occurs.

Table 11.3—The Wagner–Nelson Method To Calculate Cumulative Drug Absorption

t (h)	C ($\mu g/mL$)	$\int_0^t C \cdot dt^a$ ($\mu g/mL \cdot h$)	$C_t + k_{el} \int_0^t C \cdot dt^b$ ($\mu g/mL$)	$\dfrac{C_t + k_{el} \int_0^t C \cdot dt \times 100}{k_{el} \int_0^\infty C \cdot dt}$ (percent)
0	0	0	0	0
1	2.28	1.140	2.416	25.7
2	3.69	4.125	4.181	44.4
3	5.52	8.730	6.559	69.7
4	5.52	14.25	7.216	76.7
5	5.08	19.55	7.406	78.7
6	4.91	24.545	7.831	83.2
8	4.10	33.555	8.093	86.0
10	3.38	41.035	8.263	87.8
12	3.33	47.745	9.012	95.8
15	2.66	56.730	9.411	100.0
24	0.80	72.300	9.404	Average = 9.407
28	0.49	74.88	9.401	
32	0.31	76.48	9.411	

[a]The cumulative areas were estimated by the trapezoidal rule from the observed t and C values.
[b]The value of k_{el} estimated by the method of least squares from ln C and t in the 15–32-h range was 0.119 h.
[c]Each value in the fourth column is expressed as a percentage of the asymptotic value, 9.407, to yield the percentage absorbed shown in the fifth column.
SOURCE: Adapted with permission from reference 6.

One shortcoming of the Wagner–Nelson method is that, because the
numerator in Equation 11.21 will always eventually equal the denominator, the cumulative absorption will always eventually equal unity, or
100% (6). Even if a drug is only 10% bioavailable, the Wagner–Nelson
plot will have an asymptote of 100%. This may be confusing when considering the relative bioavailability of different forms of a drug. For example, if one generic product was actually less efficiently absorbed than
another generic product, the Wagner–Nelson plot would clearly indicate
different absorption rates (if they were different) but could be interpreted
to imply that each product was 100% absorbed.

A resolution to this problem is provided by a modification of the
Wagner–Nelson method that is based on the cumulative relative fraction
absorbed (CRFA) (7). The difference between the CRFA and the Wagner–

Nelson methods is illustrated by Equation 11.22, where A is the standard and B is the product.

$$\text{CRFA} = \frac{C_{t(B)} + k_{el(B)} \int_0^t C_{(B)}dt \times 100}{k_{el(A)} \int_0^\infty C_{(A)}dt} \tag{11.22}$$

In this equation, the numerator contains the values for the test product B, and the denominator contains the values for the standard product A. In the CRFA method, the percentage absorption versus time of a test product is plotted with reference to a standard product. Thus, if product B is actually only 50% absorbed compared with product A, then the maximum asymptotic value for Equation 11.22 will be 50%.

The Area Under the Drug Concentration Curve (AUC)

Previously, two of the three fundamental pharmacokinetic parameters that characterize the drug concentration profile in plasma, C_{max} and T_{max}, were considered. The third parameter, the area under the drug concentration versus time curve, AUC, describes how much drug is absorbed. The area under the drug concentration curve appears in virtually all pharmacokinetic reports and bioequivalence studies, and this value is required by regulatory agencies as a measure of drug absorption efficiency (8–11). The same methods of determining AUCs and converting truncated areas to complete areas after intravenous doses apply after oral or intramuscular doses. The trapezoidal determination of the areas differs in these cases only in that at time zero the drug concentration is zero, whereas in the intravenous case, the maximum value occurred at this time. Thus, after oral dosing, the first small area under the drug concentration curve is a triangle rather than a true trapezoid. Apart from this difference, the two calculations are identical for the intravenous, oral, and intramuscular cases.

Of greater interest to the pharmacokineticist are the inferences that arise from the derived expression for the area under the drug concentration curve. As described previously, the time course of the drug concentration in blood or plasma is given by

$$C = FD/V \left[(k_a/(k_a - k_{el})) \right] (e^{-k_{el}t} - e^{-k_a t}) \tag{11.23}$$

Integration of this expression between limits of zero and infinite time yields the area under the drug concentration curve

$$AUC^{0 \to \infty} = FD/Vk_{el} \qquad (11.24)$$

The equivalent expression for the area from zero to infinite time for the bolus intravenous case is

$$AUC^{0 \to \infty} = D/Vk_{el} \qquad (11.25)$$

Comparing Equations 11.24 and 11.25 shows that the two expressions are identical except for the value F, the fraction of dose absorbed.

The denominator, which is the plasma clearance, is common to both equations, but so also is the absence of the absorption rate constant k_a. This absence might be expected in the intravenous case because no absorption phase occurs. However, this phase does exist after oral or intramuscular dosing, or any dosing that involves first-order absorption, and this phase is represented by the constant k_a in Equation 11.23. However, during the integration process, the term k_a disappears. This disappearance shows that the area under the curve is affected by the elimination rate constant but is independent of the absorption rate constant. The area under the curve is unaffected by the rate of drug absorption, but the overall shape of the curve is affected. This situation is illustrated in Table 11.4. If the therapeutically effective drug concentration was above 65 µg/

Table 11.4—Plasma Profiles Obtained from Formulations with Fast, Medium, and Slow Release Rates

	Drug Concentration in Plasma (µg/mL)		
$t\ (h^{-1})$	$k_a = 3.0\ h^{-1}$	$k_a = 1.5\ h^{-1}$	$k = 0.5\ h^{-1}$
0	0	0	0
0.5	75.3	51.3	21.6
1	88.4	73.0	37.3
1.5	87.8	80.8	48.5
2	84.4	82.4	56.3
3	76.6	78.2	64.7
4	69.3	71.5	66.9
6	56.7	58.8	62.4
8	40.5	48.1	54.6
12	31.1	32.3	37.3
24	9.4	9.7	11.3
48	1.0	1.0	1.1
$AUC^{0 \to \infty}$ ($\mu g \cdot h/mL$)	1000	1000	1000

NOTE: Profiles were constructed from Equation 11.23, where FD/V was set equal to 100 µg/mL, and k_{el} equal to 0.1 h^{-1}.

mL in this instance, then the formulation that provided the slowest release would be useless (at least in this single dose example). This occurs despite the fact that the overall bioavailability, as reflected in the area under the curve, is identical in the three formulations.

The AUC is independent of k_a, but dependent on the value of k_{el}. Equation 11.24 rearranges to Equation 11.26, which shows that the overall absorption efficiency is equal to the product of k_{el} and AUC. Thus, in bioavailability studies and bioequivalency determinations, possible variations in k_{el} between subjects and between treatments must be considered because of their possible effect on the area under the plasma curve. For a true comparison of absorption efficiency, the $k_{el}\text{AUC}^{0\rightarrow\infty}$ values should be compared, as in Equation 11.26, rather than just the areas.

$$FD/V = k_{el} \cdot \text{AUC}^{0\rightarrow\infty} \tag{11.26}$$

The parameter FD/V is useful even though it often cannot be further resolved to obtain estimates of F or V separately. In Chapter 10, the AUC following intravenous dosing was described by Equation 10.16. This equation rearranges to

$$D/V = k_{el} \text{AUC}^{0\rightarrow\infty} \tag{11.27}$$

The overall absorption efficiency from an oral or intramuscular dose, compared to an intravenous standard, is determined by dividing Equation 11.26 by Equation 11.27, as in Equation 11.28.

$$\frac{(FD/V)_{(PO)}}{D/V_{(IV)}} = \frac{k_{el} \cdot \text{AUC}^{0\rightarrow\infty}_{(PO)}}{k_{el} \cdot \text{AUC}^{0\rightarrow\infty}_{(IV)}} = F \tag{11.28}$$

where PO refers to oral dose and IV refers to intravenous dose. This can be done only when the same compound is given by both routes.

On the other hand, comparison of the relative absorption efficiency of drug from two oral formulations, A and B, or perhaps between an intramuscular or rectal dose A and an oral dose B, is obtained from the ratio of Equation 11.26 for each of the two dosages:

$$\frac{(FD/V)_{(A)}}{(FD/V)_{(B)}} = \frac{k_{el}\text{AUC}^{0\rightarrow\infty}_{(A)}}{k_{el}\text{AUC}^{0\rightarrow\infty}_{(B)}} = \frac{F_{(A)}}{F_{(B)}} \tag{11.29}$$

If, for example, the ratio $F_{(A)}$ to $F_{(B)}$ was 0.9 after adjusting for possible differences in dosing, then the overall absorption efficiency from formulation A is 90% compared with formulation B. However, this comparison provides no information regarding the absolute absorption efficiency from either formulation. Formulation B may be 100% absorbed or 1% absorbed.

Absorption Lag Time

Very often, particularly with with enteric-coated dosage forms and some slowly dissolving products, a finite time period may elapse between the time of drug administration and the time that measurable drug initially appears in plasma. This lag time is frequently difficult to detect and even more difficult to measure, principally because of the relatively small number of blood samples that are generally taken during the absorption phase of a blood profile, but also because of the relatively high data variability observed during this phase.

Interpretation of the meaning of an absorption lag time is very difficult. If a lag time is not included in the interpretation of a drug-concentration profile, then prolonged absorption is reflected in a small value of k_a. If, on the other hand, a lag time is included, then prolonged absorption is reflected in a lag time and a larger value of k_a. Separating these two alternative interpretations of a drug profile is often difficult. When fitting data by nonlinear regression many of the available computer programs tend to maximize the lag time and also maximize k_a to provide a good fit to the data. This method frequently provides a better fit to the drug-concentration profile compared with the fit when lag time is not used, but in doing so provides biased estimates of these two pharmacokinetic parameters. In these situations, the lag time often must be fixed at the initial estimated value when computer fitting.

Incorporating a lag time into Equation 11.23 results in

$$C = (FD/V)[k_a/(k_a - k_{el})][e^{-k_{el}(t - t_o)} - e^{-k_a(t - t_o)}] \quad (11.30)$$

The only difference between Equations 11.23 and 11.30 is that the term t in the exponential function has been replaced by $t - t_o$.

When a lag time occurs, it can be recognized in two ways: intuitively and analytically. Intuitively, if undetectable drug levels are obtained during initial sampling periods, then a lag time exists. On the other hand, if the first sampling detects drug, but at very low levels, then whether a true lag time should be included in the absorption phase is not immediately obvious. Several possible approaches exist to resolve this dilemma. One approach will be described here.

Previously, methods were described to strip a drug concentration curve based on Equation 11.23. The treatment demonstrated that if the model was correct for the data, the intercepts of the terminal elimination slope and the residual slope on the y axis would be identical and would equal $FD/V[k_a/(k_a - k_{el})]$. This situation was illustrated in Figure 11.1.

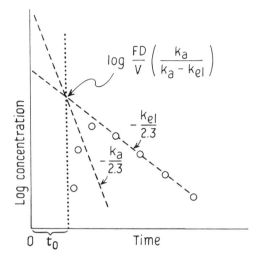

Figure 11.3. Graphical method to determine absorption lag time.

The situation when a lag time exists is illustrated in Figure 11.3. Interpretation of a drug profile by the method of residuals yields different intercepts from the extrapolated elimination and residual slopes at time zero, the time at which the dose was administered. In this case, the lag time, and also consequently the true value of FD/V, can be estimated from the point at which the two slopes intercept. Other ways exist for estimating the lag time, including direct computer analysis, but the graphical procedure is simple and accurate enough to provide initial estimates of the lag time.

Cumulative Urinary Excretion of Unchanged Drug

Equation 11.3 described the time course of the amount of drug in the body with respect to time following an oral or intramuscular dose. The rate equation for urinary recovery of unchanged drug, dA_u/dt, is found by multiplying that equation by k_e (the rate constant for urinary excretion):

$$dA_u/dt = k_e FD\{[k_a/(k_a - k_{el})]\}(e^{-k_{el}t} - e^{-k_a t}) \tag{11.31}$$

Integration of this expression yields

$$A_u = (FDk_e/k_{el})\{1 - [1/(k_a - k_{el})](k_a e^{-k_{el}t} - k_{el}e^{-k_a t})\} \tag{11.32}$$

This equation describes the cumulative urinary recovery of unchanged drug with respect to time. In this example, no absorption lag time is assumed. However, if a lag time did exist, the equation could readily be adapted simply by replacing t with $t - t_0$. Equation 11.32 can also be written as Equation 11.33, where A_u^∞ is the total urinary recovery of unchanged drug. This representation is analogous to Equation 10.27 for the intravenous case.

$$A_u = A_u^\infty = \{1 - [1/(k_a - k_{el})](k_a e^{-k_{el}t} - k_{el}e^{-k_a t})\} \tag{11.33}$$

This equation shows that at time 0 the exponential terms reduce to $k_a - k_{el}$, and therefore $A_u = 0$. On the other hand, when time increases to a very large value, or infinity, $A_u = A_u^\infty$. A cumulative urinary excretion plot can be constructed between these limits. In exactly the same way as in the intravenous case, the elimination phase of this equation is controlled by the overall elimination rate constant, k_{el}, rather than k_e, and the ratio k_e/k_{el} determines the actual quantity of drug recovered by this route, that is, $A_u^\infty = FD(k_e/k_{el})$. If all of the drug is cleared unchanged in the urine, then $k_e = k_{el}$ and $A_u^\infty = FD$. On the other hand, if all the drug is metabolized, then $k_e = 0$ and A_u will also equal zero, and no drug will be voided unchanged in the urine.

If k_a is greater than k_{el}, how might a sigma-minus plot be constructed from urinary excretion data? This situation is more complex than in the intravenous case because there are two exponents in Equations 11.32 and 11.33. Consider Equation 11.33. If k_a is greater than k_{el}, then as time increases postdose, the exponential term $e^{-k_a t}$ will approach zero quicker than the exponential term $e^{-k_{el}t}$. When that occurs, Equation 11.33 will reduce to

$$A_u = A_u^\infty\{1 - [1/(k_a - k_{el})](k_a e^{-k_{el}t})\} \tag{11.34}$$

Equation 11.34 rearranges to Equation 11.35, and in logarithmic form to Equation 11.36.

$$A_u^\infty - A_u = A_u^\infty[k_a/(k_a - k_{el})]\, e^{-k_{el}t} \tag{11.35}$$

$$\log [A_u^\infty - A_u] = \log \{A_u^\infty[k_a/(k_a - k_{el})]\} - (k_{el}/2.3)\, t \tag{11.36}$$

This equation is used to construct sigma-minus plots from urinary excretion data. If the logarithm of $A_u^\infty - A_u$, that is, the quantity of drug remaining to be excreted, is plotted against time, a slope of $-k_{el}/2.3$ and an intercept of $\log [A_u^\infty(k_a/(k_a - k_{el})]$ are obtained. This plot is illustrated in Figure 11.4. The meaning of the slope of the line and the intercept of the extrapolated line at zero time in this case is similar to the previous interpretation of drug concentration data for this model (Figure 11.1).

The numerical value of the overall elimination rate constant, k_{el}, is thus obtained from the slope of the terminal linear portion of the profile.

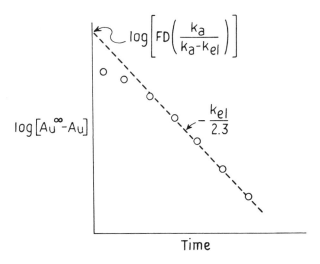

Figure 11.4. Construction of a sigma-minus plot from cumulative urinary excretion of unchanged drug.

The slope is not linear at early times postdose but appears to drop off in an inverted hockey stick shape. This effect is due to the absorption phase contributing to the profile at early times. If the value of the intercept of the straight portion of the profile, A_u^∞, and k_{el} are known, k_a can be calculated from

$$k_a = [(\text{intercept})(k_e)]/(\text{intercept} - A_u^\infty) \tag{11.37}$$

The value of k_e is obtained from the ratio A_u^∞/FD if the value of F is known. The value k_m is then obtained by subtracting k_e from k_{el}. However, if the value of F is not known, neither k_e nor k_m can be calculated. For example, if only 50% of an oral dose is recovered unchanged in the urine, distinguishing whether the other 50% is metabolized, excreted by some other route, or simply not absorbed is impossible unless intravenous data are available for comparison, or some other means is available to establish absorption efficiency.

If the flip-flop model occurs, that is, the absorption rate constant is smaller than the elimination rate constant, then the analytical procedure is identical to the procedure just described. However, the sigma-minus expression will be expressed as

$$\log (A_u^\infty - A_u) = \log \{A_u^\infty[k_{el}/(k_{el} - k_a)]\} - (k_a/2.3)\, t \tag{11.38}$$

The terminal slope will then yield k_a, and k_{el} will be obtained from

$$k_{el} = [(\text{intercept})\,(k_e)/(\text{intercept} - A_u^\infty) \tag{11.39}$$

The problem encountered here is again that of establishing which rate constant is which. Again, the best way to establish this is from intravenous data, where the elimination rate constant can be obtained independent of any absorption effect.

Urinary excretion data can be used to determine drug bioavailability in much the same way as drug concentrations in plasma, and often more effectively (12–14).

From Scheme 11.1, urinary recovery of an orally administered drug is given by

$$\text{urinary recovery} = fFD \qquad (11.40)$$

where F is the fraction of drug absorbed into the circulation, and f is the fraction of absorbed drug that is excreted unchanged in urine (k_e/k_{el}). By comparing the urinary recovery of unchanged drug from two formulations (a and b), the relationship in Equation 11.41 can be obtained.

$$A_{uA}^\infty/A_{uB}^\infty = (f_A F_A D_A)/(f_B F_B D_B) \qquad (11.41)$$

Assuming that D_A equals D_B, or at least the actual administered drug doses can be accounted for, and also $f_A = f_B$, that is, the same relationship between renal and plasma clearance is obtained with the two formulations, then Equation 11.41 reduces to

$$A_{uA}^\infty/A_{uB}^\infty - F_A/F_B \qquad (11.42)$$

From this equation the relative urinary excretion from the two formulations provides a direct measure of relative bioavailability. If formulation b is an intravenous injection, in other words, if formulation b is 100% absorbed, then F_B can be set equal to unity, and the ratio of urinary recovery from the test formulation and the intravenous dose yields F, the absolute absorption efficiency.

Instead of measuring urinary recovery of unchanged drug, measuring recovery of a metabolite can work just as well. This approach has been used, for example, to determine griseofulvin absorption efficacy by measuring the urinary recovery of the major metabolite, desmethylgriseofulvin. In this case, urinary recovery is related to absorbed drug as in Equation 11.43, where f' is the fraction of drug excreted as the metabolite (k_m/k_{el}).

$$M_{uA}^\infty/M_{uB}^\infty (f_A' F_A D_A)/(f_B' F_B D_B) \qquad (11.43)$$

Summary

1. Absorption of drug into the systemic circulation from the GI tract is a complex phenomenon. Interpretation of absorption as a first-order process is usually a simplification.

2. The apparent absorption rate constant is a function of loss of drug from the absorption site by all processes.

3. Correct interpretation of drug concentration profile in plasma depends on the relative value of the absorption rate constant, which may be greater than, equal to, or less than the elimination rate constant.

4. Estimates of rate constants can be made by curve stripping procedures, or residuals.

5. Drug absorption rates can be obtained from plasma data, independent of elimination rates, using the Wagner–Nelson method for the one-compartment model, or the Loo–Riegelman method for the two-compartment model. An alternative method is based on cumulative relative fraction absorbed (CRFA).

6. The area under the drug profile in plasma can be used to determine relative bioavailability, or absolute absorption efficiency, of an orally dosed drug.

7. For a drug whose absorption is delayed, incorporation of an absorption lag time is necessary to obtain accurate estimates of the absorption rate constant.

8. Sigma-minus plots from urinary excretion data provide estimates of rate constants for drug absorption, excretion, and metabolism.

Literature Cited

1. Viswanathan, C. T.; Booker, H. E.; Welling, P. G. *J. Clin. Pharm.*, **1978**, *18*, 100–105.
2. Patel, R. B.; Welling, P. G. *J. Pharm. Sci*, **1982**, *71*, 529–532.
3. Robinson, J. R.; Goshman, L. M. In *Pharmaceutics and Pharmacy Practice*, Banker, G. S.; Chalmers, R. K., Eds. Lippincott: Philadelphia, 1982, p 320.
4. Wagner, J. G.; Nelson, E. *J. Pharm. Sci.*, **1964**, *53*, 1392–1394.
5. Loo, J. C. K.; Riegelman, S. *J. Pharm. Sci.*, **1968**, *57*, 918–928.
6. Wagner, J. G. *Fundamentals of Clinical Pharmacokinetics.* Intelligence Publications: Hamilton, IL, 1975, p 171.
7. Welling, P. G.; Patel, R. B.; Patel, U. R.; Gillespie, W.R.; Craig, W. A.; Albert, K. S. *J. Pharm. Sci.*, **1982**, *71*, 1259–1263.
8. *Guidelines for Biopharmaceutical Studies in Man*; American Pharmaceutical Association, Academy of Pharmaceutical Sciences: Washington, DC, 1972; Appendix I, p 17.

9. Skelly, J. P. *Bioavailability Policies and Guidelines*, 13th Annual International Industrial Pharmacy Conference, Austin, TX, 1974.
10. Chasseaud, L. F.; Taylor, T. *Ann. Rev. Pharmacol*, **1974**, *14*, 35–46.
11. *Fed. Reg.* **1977**, *45*, 1634.
12. Kwan, K. C.; Till, A. E. *J. Pharm. Sci.*, **1973**, *62*, 1494–1497.
13. Wagner, J. G. *J. Pharm. Sci.*, **1967**, *56*, 489–494.
14. Glazko, A. J.; Kinlel, A. W.; Alegnani, W. C.; Holmes, G. L. *Clin. Pharmacol. Ther.*, **1968**, *9*, 472–483.

Problems

1. A 500-mg dose of the sulfonamide sulfamethoxazole is administered as an oral tablet to a human subject. Eighty percent of the drug is absorbed, and the balance is excreted unchanged in feces. The drug distributes into an apparently homogeneous body volume of 12 L, and has an absorption half-life of 15 min and an overall elimination half-life of 12 h. Calculate the following: (i) $AUC^{0\rightarrow\infty}$, (ii) C_{max}, and (iii) T_{max}.

2. Recalculate the values in problem 1 if all parameter values remained unchanged, but the elimination half-life was increased to 18 hours.

3. In a controlled, crossover bioavailability study of oral dosage forms, formulation *A*, containing 250 mg of a drug, was tested against formulation B, containing 150 mg of the same drug. The drug is extensively metabolized in the body to one major metabolite. Urinary recovery of the metabolite was 215 mg from formulation A and 145 mg from formulation B. Calculate the ratio of availability from formulation A to availability from formulation B.

4. After 200 mg of a drug is administered orally, 50% is absorbed into the circulation. The drug has a first-order absorption rate constant of $2.0\ h^{-1}$ and is eliminated from the body in equal proportions by metabolism and by excretion in unchanged form in urine. The overall biological half-life is 3.46 h. If a sigma-minus plot were constructed from the urinary excretion data, what would be the values of (a) the rate constant from the slope of the line, and (b) the intercept of the line on the y ordinate ($t = 0$)?

5. A patient receives a drug dose of 500 mg orally. Only 80% of the drug is absorbed from the GI tract, and the balance is excreted unchanged in the feces. The drug is not appreciably bound to plasma proteins and, of the absorbed drug, 25% is metabolized and 75% is excreted as unchanged drug by the kidneys. The following drug concentrations were obtained after a single dose:

Time (h)	Concentration ($\mu g/mL$)
0.0	0.0
0.25	6.1
0.5	10.0
1	13.8
2	14.3
4	10.3
8	4.7
12	2.1
24	0.2

Calculate the following: (i) k_{el}, (ii) $t_{1/2}$, (iii) k_a, (iv) $t_{1/2 \ (abs)}$, (v) distribution volume, and (vi) plasma clearance.

6. From the data in problem 5, construct a plot of cumulative excretion of drug (mg) in urine. Use Cartesian coordinate graph paper and the same time intervals as for the drug concentration in plasma data. Calculate: (i) k_{el}, (ii) k_e, and (iii) k_m. Are these values the same as from the plasma data?

7. From the data in problems 5 and 6, calculate the renal clearance. Why is the renal clearance different from the plasma clearance?

12

Multiple-Dose Kinetics

Most drug therapy involves repeated administration of separate doses over a variable period. It is in this aspect of drug therapy that a knowledge of pharmacokinetics plays a particularly important role. Factors that are important to know are how long therapy should be continued, whether a few days for an antibiotic or prolonged periods for an antidiabetic or hypotensive agent; how frequently a drug should be given to achieve the optimum blood-level profile; what type of accumulation, if any, will occur with repeated doses; and how long it will take for steady-state levels to be achieved (1).

Drug Accumulation with Repeated Doses

The treatment in this chapter is based on simple one-compartment and first-order kinetics and assumes that drug is given by multiple intravenous bolus injections. Nonetheless, provided that the kinetics are first-order and linear, conclusions drawn from the intravenous bolus approach apply to other dosage routes that may involve repeated intravenous infusion, multiple oral or intramuscular doses, or any other means of drug administration (2–4). Another assumption is that the drug is given at equally spaced intervals, which may not apply in practice; the more irregular the drug intervals, the more difficult characterization or prediction of the accumulation and steady-state drug profile will be. Computer programs are available for blood-level analysis in this type of situation. However, this and all other variations in drug administration are

0065-7719/86/0185-0187$06.00/1

based on the principle of drug accumulation resulting from regularly spaced dosing intervals, which is described here.

In Chapter 10, the quantity of drug in the body following bolus intravenous injection was described by Equation 10.1, where the initial amount of drug in the body, A_0, is equal to the dose, and k_{el} is the elimination rate constant.

$$A = A_0 e^{-k_{el}t} = De^{-k_{el}t} \qquad (12.1)$$

If a certain time period, τ, is allowed to elapse after the dose, then the amount of drug in the body, $A_{1(min)}$, is given by

$$A_{1(min)} = De^{-k_{el}\tau} \qquad (12.2)$$

If τ is sufficiently long, that is, longer than 4.5 drug half-lives, then A will approach zero at time τ. However, if τ is not long compared to the drug half-life, then A at time τ will be less than D but greater than zero. If another dose is added at time τ, then the amount of drug in the body $A_{2(max)}$ will equal that amount remaining from the previous dose plus the new dose:

$$A_{2(max)} = De^{-k_{el}\tau} + D = D(1 + e^{-k_{el}\tau}) \qquad (12.3)$$

At the end of another time interval τ, the quantity of drug remaining in the body, $A_{2(min)}$, will be described by

$$A_{2(min)} = D(1 + e^{-k_{el}\tau})e^{-k_{el}\tau} = D(e^{-k_{el}\tau} + e^{-2k_{el}\tau}) \qquad (12.4)$$

This process can be repeated with more doses so that expressions for $A_{n(max)}$ and $A_{n(min)}$ can be written after each dose and each dosage interval, where n is the number of doses. From Equations 12.3 and 12.4, the general Equations 12.5 and 12.6 can be written to describe the maximum and minimum quantities of drug in the body following n doses.

$$A_{n(max)} = D(1 + e^{-k_{el}\tau} \ldots + e^{-(n-1)k_{el}\tau}) \qquad (12.5)$$

$$A_{n(min)} = D(e^{-k_{el}\tau} + e^{-2k_{el}\tau} \ldots + e^{-nk_{el}\tau}) \qquad (12.6)$$

These expressions become unwieldly as additional doses are added. To obtain more simple expressions, Equations 12.5 and 12.6 can be written in shorthand form as Equations 12.7 and 12.8, respectively.

$$A_{n(max)} = D \cdot X \qquad (12.7)$$

$$A_{n(min)} = D \cdot Xe^{-k_{el}\tau} \qquad (12.8)$$

In these equations, the quantity X is equal to the entire parenthetical term in Equation 12.5.

If Equation 12.8 is subtracted from Equation 12.7, Equation 12.9 is obtained.

$$A_{n(max)} - A_{n(min)} = DX(1 - e^{-k_{el}\tau}) \qquad (12.9)$$

Subtraction of Equation 12.6 from Equation 12.5 yields Equation 12.10.

$$A_{n(max)} - A_{n(min)} = D(1 - e^{-nk_{el}\tau}) \qquad (12.10)$$

The left side of Equation 12.10 is identical to the left side of Equation 12.9; therefore, Equation 12.11 can be written, and this equation reduces to Equation 12.12.

$$DX(1 - e^{-k_{el}\tau}) = D(1 - e^{-nk_{el}\tau}) \qquad (12.11)$$

$$X = (1 - e^{-nk_{el}\tau})/(1 - e^{-k_{el}\tau}) \qquad (12.12)$$

Equation 12.12 is a short and manageable form of shorthand notation that can be substituted into Equations 12.7 and 12.8 to obtain Equations 12.13 and 12.14.

$$A_{n(max)} = D(1 - e^{-nk_{el}\tau})/(1 - e^{-k_{el}\tau}) \qquad (12.13)$$

$$A_{n(min)} = D(1 - e^{-nk_{el}\tau}) e^{-k_{el}\tau}/(1 - e^{-k_{el}\tau}) \qquad (12.14)$$

These two expressions are general terms that describe the maximum and minimum amounts of drug in the body after n doses.

A third expression, Equation 12.15, can now be written to describe the quantity of drug in the body at any time during a dosage interval, where the term t is the time elapsed since the last dose.

$$A_{n(t)} = D(1 - e^{-nk_{el}\tau}) e^{-k_{el}t}/(1 - e^{-k_{el}\tau}) \qquad (12.15)$$

Three equations, 12.13, 12.14, and 12.15, have now been derived in terms of amounts of drug. These expressions can be converted to concentration terms simply by dividing both sides of the equations by the distribution volume, V, to give Equations 12.16, 12.17, and 12.18.

$$C_{n(max)} = D(1 - e^{-nk_{el}\tau})/V(1 - e^{-k_{el}\tau}) \qquad (12.16)$$

$$C_{n(min)} = D(1 - e^{-nk_{el}\tau}) e^{-k_{el}\tau}/V(1 - e^{-k_{el}\tau}) \qquad (12.17)$$

$$C_{n(t)} = D(1 - e^{-nk_{el}\tau}) e^{-k_{el}t}/V(1 - e^{-k_{el}\tau}) \qquad (12.18)$$

These expressions describe the concentration of drug, C, in the body in blood, plasma, or serum during repeated dosing. If dosing is continued, accumulation will continue until eventually the rate of drug elimination will equal the rate of drug administration, and steady state will be achieved. Steady state will continue indefinitely, provided the drug dosage and elimination rate remain constant. Thus, the drug concentration can be expanded to infinity. Equations 12.16, 12.17, and 12.18 can be rewritten with n equal to ∞ as in Equations 12.19, 12.20, and 12.21.

$$C_{\infty(max)} = D/V(1 - e^{-k_{el}\tau}) \tag{12.19}$$

$$C_{\infty(min)} = De^{-k_{el}\tau}/V(1 - e^{-k_{el}\tau}) \tag{12.20}$$

$$C_{\infty(t)} = De^{-k_{el}t}/V(1 - e^{-k_{el}\tau}) \tag{12.21}$$

Equations 12.19, 12.20, and 12.21 describe the maximum, minimum, and intermediate drug concentrations, respectively, at steady state for a given dose, distribution volume, elimination rate constant, and dosage interval.

The pattern of drug accumulation and steady state $C_{\infty(max)}$ and $C_{\infty(min)}$ values during repeated intravenous bolus injections at intervals of τ h is illustrated in Figure 12.1.

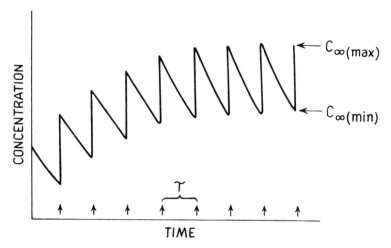

Figure 12.1. Drug concentrations during multiple intravenous injections, during the accumulation phase, and at steady state.

Having been defined, $C_{\infty(max)}$, $C_{\infty(min)}$, and $C_{\infty(t)}$ can now be used to demonstrate some basic rules regarding multiple-dose kinetics. For example, knowing to what extent drug concentrations oscillate between maximum and minimum values at steady state is often important. How wide apart are the peaks and troughs? This difference can be determined simply by subtracting $C_{\infty(min)}$ from $C_{\infty(max)}$ as in Equation 12.22.

$$C_{\infty(max)} - C_{\infty(min)} = \frac{D}{V(1 - e^{-k_{el}\tau})} - \frac{De^{-k_{el}\tau}}{V(1 - e^{-k_{el}\tau})} \qquad (12.22)$$

$$= \frac{D(1 - e^{-k_{el}\tau})}{V(1 - e^{-k_{el}\tau})} = \frac{D}{V} = C_0$$

This equation shows that the difference between the maximum and minimum concentrations at steady state is identical to the maximum concentration obtained after the initial dose, C_0. This identity applies whether the drug is given by intravenous injection, orally, or by any other dosage route. This relationship is not that remarkable. With each successive dose, a certain concentration of drug is added to the concentration remaining from the previous dose. The drug concentration preceding the initial dose is zero. However, if a maximum drug concentration of 10 µg/mL is obtained following an initial dose of a drug, then, regardless of the extent of accumulation, the maximum drug concentration in plasma will always be 10 µg/mL greater than the minimum drug concentration at steady state.

Equation 12.21 describes the drug concentration at any time t during a dosage interval at steady state. If that expression is integrated between the limits $t = 0$ and $t = \tau$ during a dosage interval at steady state, Equation 12.23 is obtained.

$$\int_0^\tau \frac{De^{-k_{el}t}}{V(1 - e^{-k_{el}\tau})} \, dt = \frac{D}{V(1 - e^{-k_{el}\tau})} \int_0^\tau e^{-k_{el}t} \, dt = D/Vk_{el} = AUC^{0\to\tau}$$

$$(12.23)$$

This expression describes the area under the drug-concentration curve during a dosage interval, τ, and is identical to the expression for the area under the drug concentration curve from zero to infinite time following a single intravenous dose (Equation 10.16). Thus, the area under the curve during a dosage interval at steady state from a multiple-dose regimen is equal to the area to infinite time following a single dose, provided that the same dose is administered, and the kinetics is unchanged during multiple doses. This situation is illustrated in Figure 12.2 and applies equally to oral and intravenous dosing. The only difference is that in the oral case, the area expression must contain the parameter F, the fraction of dose absorbed into the systemic circulation.

Because of the identity between the single dose and steady-state areas, the plasma clearance, Vk_{el}, can readily be obtained from multiple dose data just as from single dose data, by dividing the dose by the appropriate area under the plasma curve. The steady-state area can be

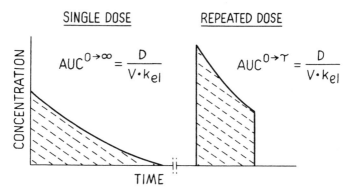

Figure 12.2. Areas under drug concentration versus time profiles in plasma follow-ing a single dose, and at steady state following multiple doses.

used also to determine whether any changes occur in the pharmacokinetic behavior of a drug during multiple dosing. For example, if the multiple-dose area from zero to τ is less than the single-dose area from zero to infinite time (or less than one would predict from the single-dose area), then this difference may be evidence of enzyme induction or of an in-creased distribution volume with repeated doses. On the other hand, if the repeated dose area is greater than the single dose area, then this may be evidence of drug-metabolizing enzyme inhibition or of reduction in the distribution volume. After oral doses, drug bioavailability may be altered during multiple doses because of saturable absorption, increased GI degradation, altered GI physiology (perhaps due to the drug), or altered first-pass metabolism associated with enzyme induction or inhi-bition.

Although the steady-state area is obtained during a dosage interval, Equation 12.23 does not contain the value . This indicates that the identity between the steady-state zero to τ area and the single-dose zero to infinity area remains the same, regardless of the dosage interval. How frequently or infrequently drug is given is not important.

A parameter that is used frequently in multiple-dose kinetics is the expression for the mean drug concentration at steady state, $\overline{C}_\infty$. This expression was first described by Wagner et al. in 1965 (5) and is readily obtained by dividing Equation 12.23 by the dosing interval τ, to yield

$$\overline{C}_\infty = D/Vk_{el}\tau \qquad (12.24)$$

This expression is valid for both intravenous and oral doses and has some interesting properties in the oral case (6). However, until the oral case is considered in detail, Equation 12.24 may be considered as a universal form of description of mean steady-state drug levels between $C_{\infty(max)}$ and $C_{\infty(min)}$.

Drug Accumulation Rate

Important questions that arise when considering drug accumulation with repeated doses are how fast and how much. How long does it take for drug concentrations in plasma to reach or approach steady-state values, and to what extent will levels increase during that time?

Answers to those questions will be based on Equations 12.16 and 12.19 for C_{max}. Dividing Equation 12.16 by Equation 12.19 and cancelling like terms yields

$$C_{n(max)}/C_{\infty(max)} = 1 - e^{-k_{el}\tau} \tag{12.25}$$

This equation can be revised and simplified to obtain a more general expression relating the frequency of drug dosing and half-life. Because k_{el} equals $\ln 2/t_{1/2}$, Equation 12.25 can be written as Equation 12.26, in which $t_{1/2}$ is the drug elimination half-life.

$$C_{n(max)}/C_{\infty(max)} = 1 - e^{-n\cdot\ln 2\cdot\tau/t_{1/2}} \tag{12.26}$$

Because $e^{\ln 2} = 2$ in the same way that $10^{\log_{10} 2} = 2$, Equation 12.26 rearranges to

$$C_{n(max)}/C_{\infty(max)} = 1 - 2^{-n\tau/t_{1/2}} \tag{12.27}$$

If the ratio $\tau/t_{1/2}$ is expressed as a single parameter, ϵ, then Equation 12.27 can be written as

$$C_{n(max)}/C_{\infty(max)} = 1 - 2^{-n\epsilon} \tag{12.28}$$

This expression is useful because of its general application; it is dependent only on the relationship between how often a drug is administered and the drug half-life. How can the number of doses required to reach 95% of steady state during a repeated dose regimen be determined, that is, when does $C_{n(max)}/C_{\infty(max)}$ equal 95%?

Consider three different situations. In the first situation, drug is administered each half-life; in the second situation, once every two half-lives; and in the third situation, twice every half-life. The calculations are summarized in Figure 12.3.

The first situation happens quite frequently. For example, doxycycline has a half-life of about 10–12 h and is frequently dosed twice daily.

If the drug is dosed every half-life, then from Figure 12.3, $\epsilon = 1$ and $n = 4.35$. These values may be interpreted to mean that 95% of steady state is not reached at the fourth dose but is exceeded at the fifth dose.

$$\frac{C_{n(max)}}{C_{\infty(max)}} = 95\%$$

SITUATION 1	SITUATION 2	SITUATION 3
$\tau = t_{1/2}, \; \varepsilon = 1$	$\tau = 2(t_{1/2}), \; \varepsilon = 2$	$\tau = 0.5(t_{1/2}), \; \varepsilon = 0.5$
$1 - 2^{-n\varepsilon} = 0.95$	$2^{2n} = 20$	$2^{0.5n} = 20$
$2^{-n\varepsilon} = 0.05$	$n = 2.17$ DOSES	$n = 8.7$ DOSES
$2^{-n} = 0.05$		
$2^{n} = 20$		
$n = 4.35$ DOSES		

Figure 12.3. Calculations to obtain the number of doses required to reach 95% of steady state during a multiple-dose regimen.

The second situation is also common and applies to drugs such as the aminoglycosides that have half-lives of 3–4 h and are commonly dosed at 6–8-h intervals. In this situation, $\epsilon = 2$, and only 2.17 doses are required to reach 95% of steady state. The number of doses in this situation is only one-half the number of doses required when $\epsilon = 1$.

The third situation is when the drug is administered twice every half-life, and applies to such drugs as digoxin, which has a half-life of about 2 days and is generally dosed once each day. In this situation, $\epsilon = 0.5$, and the number of doses required to reach 95% of steady state increases to 8.7, which is double the value in the first situation.

The number of doses required to reach 95% of steady-state drug levels is thus directly related to dosing frequency. However, despite the different number of doses required in each of the three situations, the time taken to reach 95% of steady state is identical. If the half-life of a drug were 10 h, then in all three situations described previously, approximately 44 h would be needed to reach 95% of steady state. Therefore, just as in the intravenous infusion case discussed in Chapter 10, the time required to approach steady state during a multiple-dosage regimen is independent of the dosage frequency, or input rate, and is dependent solely on the elimination half-life of the drug. If a drug has a half-life of

24 h, then 4.4 days would be needed to reach 95% of steady state, no matter how frequently the drug is administered.

The Degree of Drug Accumulation with Repeated Dosing and the Loading Dose Required To Instantaneously Achieve Steady-State Levels

The degree to which drug levels accumulate with multiple doses can be expressed in terms of the ratio $C_{\infty(max)}/C_{1(max)}$, or Equation 12.19 divided by D/V, as in

$$\frac{C_{\infty(max)}}{C_{1(max)}} = R = \frac{\dfrac{D}{V(1 - e^{-k_{el}\tau})}}{\dfrac{D}{V}} = \frac{1}{1 - e^{-k_{el}\tau}} \tag{12.29}$$

In this equation, R represents $C_{\infty(max)}/C_{1(max)}$. This function can be rewritten as Equation 12.30 after making the same substitutions as those used to obtain Equation 12.28.

$$R = 1/(1 - 2^{-\epsilon}) \tag{12.30}$$

where ϵ again represents the ratio $\tau/t_{1/2}$. In Table 12.1, five representative values of R are described where $\epsilon = 0.25, 0.5, 1, 2$, and 4, (i.e., the drug is given four times, twice, once, every second, and every fourth half-life, respectively). If a drug is given once every half-life, steady-state drug concentrations in plasma will be double those achieved after the initial dose. If the dosing frequency is increased to twice every half-life, then the accumulation factor is increased to 3.4. If the dosing frequency is reduced so that one dose is given every second half-life, the accumulation factor is reduced to only 1.3. The two additional values in the table show the more extreme cases in which dosing four times every half-life results in over sixfold accumulation, while dosing once every four drug elimination half-lives results in essentially zero accumulation. The latter of these two examples is a typical case in which drug levels from the initial dose decline to zero before the next dose is given. This common situation occurs with many penicillins and cephalosporins that have half-lives of approximately 1 h and are commonly dosed every 4–6 h. Drug accumulation cannot possibly occur, and repeated doses yield the same drug concentrations as the first dose.

The types of drug profiles obtained with the three situations where $\epsilon = 0.5, 1$, or 2 are shown in Figure 12.4. The time to reach steady state is identical in each case.

Just as in the infusion case described in Chapter 10, drugs that have

Table 12.1—Extent of Drug Accumulation R with Multiple Dosing

ϵ	R
0.25	6.3
0.5	3.4
1	2.0
2	1.33
4	1.07

NOTE: values were calculated from Equation 12.30. See text for explanation of symbols.

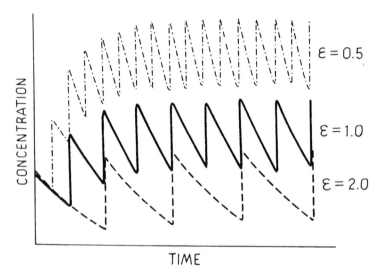

Figure 12.4. *Drug profiles obtained following multiple intravenous doses of a drug administered at intervals of 1/2, 1, and 2 half-lives.*

long elimination half-lives lead to slow accumulation. For these compounds, administering some type of loading dose to achieve therapeutic steady-state levels quickly may be necessary. By judicious borrowing from the infusion concepts, and appreciating that the overall kinetics of drug accumulation and decline are identical in that situation and the one now presented, if an initial loading dose comprises the same quantity of drug that is in the body at steady state, then the required steady-state drug level will be achieved with the initial dose and will be maintained by the subsequent doses. From Table 12.1, if a drug is given every half-life, then the accumulation factor is 2, and the required loading dose to achieve steady-state levels immediately is twice the maintenance dose. If the drug is given twice every half-life, the loading dose is 3.4 times the maintenance dose. If the dose is given once every four half-lives ($\epsilon = 4$), then no loading dose is required because of negligible drug accumulation.

First-Order Absorption Case

The preceding discussions are based on multiple intravenous bolus injections. However, all of the conclusions regarding drug accumulation and its time dependency apply equally when the drug is given orally or by any other route.

Some additional aspects of multiple oral dosing need to be understood before leaving this subject. The terms for $C_{\infty(max)}$, $C_{\infty(min)}$, and $\overline{C}_{\infty}$ for the oral or first-order absorption case are given by Equations 12.31, 12.32, and 12.33, respectively.

$$C_{\infty(max)} = \frac{FD}{V}\left[\frac{1}{1 - e^{-k_{el}\tau}}\right]\left[\frac{k_a(1 - e^{-k_{el}\tau})}{k_{el}(1 - e^{-k_a})}\right]^{k_{el}/k_a - k_{el}} \tag{12.31}$$

$$C_{\infty(min)} = \frac{FD}{V}\left[\frac{k_a}{k_a - k_{el}}\right]\left[\frac{e^{-k_{el}\tau}}{1 - e^{-k_{el}}} - \frac{e^{-k_a\tau}}{1 - e^{-k_a\tau}}\right] \tag{12.32}$$

$$\overline{C}_{\infty} = FD/Vk_{el}\tau \tag{12.33}$$

The increased complexity of Equations 12.31 and 12.32 is due to the presence of the absorption rate constant k_a. The first-order absorption phase has the effect of reducing $C_{\infty(max)}$ and increasing $C_{\infty(min)}$. This effect is observed by comparing the $C_{\infty(max)}$ values from Equations 12.20 and 12.31 and the $C_{\infty(min)}$ values from Equations 12.21 and 12.32. In the first-order absorption case a flatter drug profile (i.e., a lower $C_{\infty(max)}$ and a higher $C_{\infty(min)}$ value) is obtained with decreasing values of k_a. However, from Equation 12.33 the value $\overline{C}_{\infty}$, the mean drug level, is independent of k_a. Except for the presence of the function F, the fraction of the dose absorbed, Equation 12.33 is identical to the intravenous Equation 12.24. $C_{\infty(max)}$ and $C_{\infty(min)}$ are markedly dependent on the magnitude of k_a, while $\overline{C}_{\infty}$ is unaffected. This situation is depicted in Figure 12.5. If the absorption rate constant were reduced to the point where the absorption efficiency, F, was reduced, then the whole drug profile including $\overline{C}_{\infty}$ would be reduced. Multiplying Equation 12.33 by the value τ yields the area under the drug concentration curve shown in Equation 12.34.

$$AUC^{0\rightarrow\tau} = FD/Vk_{el} \tag{12.34}$$

Except for the F value, which accompanies all oral dosing, Equation 12.34 is identical to Equation 12.23 for the intravenous case. Just as in the case of the area from zero to infinite time after single doses, the area from time zero to τ at steady state during repeated doses is independent of the absorption rate constant.

The last parameter to consider is the time at which peak or maximum drug levels, $T_{\infty(max)}$, occur after repeated oral dosing at steady state. In the

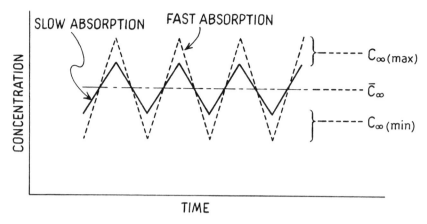

Figure 12.5. Values of $C_{\infty(max)}$, $C_{\infty(min)}$, and $\overline{C}_\infty$ for a drug that is absorbed at a fast or slow first-order rate.

intravenous case, the $T_{\infty(max)}$ occurs immediately after each dose. However, in the first order absorption case, the value $T_{\infty(max)}$ is given by Equation 12.35.

$$T_{\infty(max)} = \frac{1}{k_a - k_{el}} \ln \left[\frac{k_a(1 - e^{-k_{el}\tau})}{k_{el}(1 - e^{-k_a\tau})} \right] \tag{12.35}$$

This equation is similar to the expression for T_{max} following a single dose (Chapter 11) except for the logarithmic function. The value $T_{\infty(max)}$, relative to the last dose, is always shorter than the time T_{max} after a single dose.

Consider a drug that has an absorption rate constant, k_a, of 1 h^{-1} and an elimination rate constant, k_{el}, of 0.1 h^{-1}, and that the drug is dosed every 6 h. After the first dose, according to Equation 11.19, T_{max} occurs at 2.6 h, or 2 h and 36 min after dosing. If the drug is dosed every 6 h to reach steady state, then according to Equation 12.35, $T_{\infty(max)}$ is 1.7 h, or 1 h and 42 min. This value is almost 1 h earlier than after the single dose. Thus, if T_{max} occurred at 2.6 h after a single dose, and a blood sample was taken at 2.6 h after a dose at steady state to examine $C_{\infty(max)}$, then the sample would have been taken almost one hour too late. The peak would have been missed, the sample would have been taken when drug concentrations were in the declining postpeak phase, and $C_{\infty(max)}$ would be underestimated.

Summary

1. The extent of drug accumulation during repeated doses depends upon both the dose and the frequency with which it is administered. The rate of drug accumulation, on the other hand, depends

exclusively on the drug elimination rate constant and is independent of the dose or dosage interval.

2. Whereas $C_{\infty(max)}$ and $C_{\infty(min)}$ in the first-order absorption case are both sensitive to the value of the absorption rate constant k_a, $\overline{C}_\infty$ is independent of the absorption rate constant provided the overall bioavailability is unaffected.

3. The time of peak drug levels occurs earlier after multiple dosing compared to single dosing, and this could give rise to underestimation of the degree of drug accumulation with repeated doses.

Literature Cited

1. Kruger-Thiemer, E.; Bunger, P. *Chemotherapia*, **1965**, *10*, 61–74.
2. Wagner, J. G. *J. Clin. Pharmacol.*, **1967**, *7*, 84–88.
3. Kaplan, S. A.; Jack, M. L.; Alexander, K.; Weinfeld, R. E. *J. Pharm. Sci.*, **1971**, *62*, 1789–1796.
4. Alexanderson, B. *Eur. J. Clin. Pharmacol.*, **1972**, *4*, 82–91.
5. Wagner, J. G.; Northam, J. I.; Alway, C. D.; Carpenter, O. S. *Nature*, **1965**, *207*, 1301–1302.
6. Perrier, D.; Gibaldi, M. *J. Pharmacokinet. Biopharm.*, **1973**, *1*, 17–22.

Problems

1. A drug (100 mg) is administered to a 70-kg male patient by multiple IV injections at 6-h intervals. The drug is water-soluble and has a distribution volume equivalent to that of total body water. The drug has a biological half-life of 6 h. Calculate (i) C_{max}(initial), (ii) $C_{\infty(max)}$, (iii) $C_{\infty(min)}$, and (iv) $\overline{C}_\infty$.

2. Because of a deterioration in the patient's condition, the dose described in problem 1 has to be increased to 150 mg every 4 h. Dosing is continued until a new steady state is reached. Calculate (i) $C_{\infty(max)}$, (ii) $C_{\infty(min)}$, and (iii) C_∞.

3. A drug (100 mg) is administered to a 70-kg male patient by repeated bolus IV injections. The drug has a distribution volume of 5 L and a biological half-life of 8 h, and is injected at intervals of 8 h. Calculate the following:

   (i) $C_{\infty(max)}$
   (ii) The number of doses required to reach 95% of the steady-state concentration.
   (iii) The time necessary to reach 95% of the steady-state concentration.

4. Recalculate problem 3 if the same quantity of drug is administered to the same patient every 4 h.

5. Recalculate problem 3 if the same drug is dosed IV every 8 h to a patient with renal failure in whom the drug has a biological half-life of 20 h (volume of distribution is 5 L).

6. How would the dose be adjusted so that the same $\overline{C}_x$ can be obtained for the patient in problem 5 as was obtained for the patient in problem 3 without changing the dosage interval?

7. If the physician decided to give the same quantity of drug as in problem 3 to the patient in problem 6, at what dosing interval would it have to be given to yield the same $\overline{C}_x$ value as that for the patient in problem 3?

8. Calculate the loading dose required for the patient in problem 7 to give the $C_{x(max)}$ value instantaneously with the first dose.

9. A 500-mg oral dose of a drug is administered to a patient. Pharmacokinetic analysis yielded a first-order absorption rate constant of 0.8 h^{-1} and a first-order elimination rate constant of 0.08 h^{-1}. Calculate the following:

(i) T_{max} following the single dose

(ii) $T_{x(max)}$ at steady state if the drug was given as repeated doses at 8-h intervals.

13

Metabolite Pharmacokinetics

The pharmacokinetic treatments in Chapters 10–12 concerned the pharmacokinetics of an administered drug. Many drug metabolites are pharmacologically inactive so that, for the most part, their pharmacokinetics is relatively unimportant; however, many exceptions exist. For example, the major metabolite of procainamide, N-acetylprocainamide, has similar cardiac potency to the parent drug. Desmethyldiazepam and desmethylmethsuximide are both pharmacologically active metabolites of the parent drugs diazepam and methsuximide. Some other examples of active drug metabolites are given in Table 13.1. These examples are just a few of many active drug metabolites. In these situations it is just as important to understand the pharmacokinetics of the active metabolite as those of the parent drug.

In other situations, blood or urine concentrations of parent drug may be too low to detect or measure accurately so that attention has to be diverted to measurement of major metabolites in order to understand the phamacokinetics of the parent compound. An example of this is the antimicotic agent griseofulvin, which is rapidly metabolized in the body to desmethylgriseofulvin. Urinary excretion of this metabolite has been used as an indicator of absorption efficiency of griseofulvin.

Pharmacokinetics of Metabolite Formation and Elimination

Thus, for several different reasons, it is important to examine and understand the pharmacokinetic characteristics of a metabolite in addition to or instead of those of the parent drug. From a pharmacokinetic view-

0065-7719/86/0185-0201$06.00/1
© 1986 American Chemical Society

point, formation of a metabolite from a parent drug, and subsequent further metabolism or excretion of the metabolite, can be considered in terms of catenary chain kinetics, which is a sequence of kinetic steps in the form of A → B → C, etc.

Table 13.1—Some Pharmacologically Active Metabolites

Parent Drug	Active Metabolites
Acetylsalicylic acid	Salicylic acid
Amitriptyline	Nortriptyline
Codeine	Morphine
Flurazepam	Desalkylflurazepam
Meperidine	Normeperidine
Methamphetamine	Amphetamine
Phenacetin	Acetaminophen
Prednisone	Prednisolone
Spironolactone	Canrenone
Trimethadione	Dimethadione

Catenary chain kinetics will be considered using a simple model of an intravenously administered drug that is partially cleared via the urine in unchanged form and partially converted to a single metabolite that is subsequently excreted in urine. The simplifying assumption also will be made that the biotransformation step from drug to metabolite is first-order. Because metabolic processes are enzymatic, all metabolic steps are saturable at some drug (substrate) concentration, and some examples of this will be discussed in Chapter 16. However, the present argument will assume that the drug concentration is below that level where saturable, or Michaelis–Menten-type, kinetics becomes important, and the first-order kinetic approximation can be used. This assumption is reasonable because only a small number of drugs have exhibited saturable kinetics in the therapeutic concentration range.

The model to be used is shown in Scheme 13.1. This simple situation will illustrate some of the inherent problems associated with analysis and interpretation of these types of data. Interpretation of the data for the parent drug presents no significant problems as discussed in Chapter 10. To recapitulate from that chapter, the time course of the amount of drug in the body can be described by·

$$A = A_0 e^{-k_{el}t} \qquad (13.1)$$

where A_0 is the administered dose, t is the time elapsed since administering the drug, A is the amount of drug in the body at time t, and k_{el} is

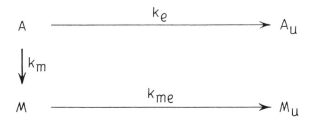

Scheme 13.1. *Kinetic scheme for intravenous drug administration and formation of a single metabolite; A is the amount of drug in body, M is the amount of metabolite in body, A_u is the cumulative amount of drug voided in urine, M_u is the cumulative amount of metabolite voided in urine, k_m is the first-order rate constant for formation of metabolite, and k_e and k_{me} are first-order rate constants for urinary excretion of drug and metabolite, respectively.*

the first-order rate constant for drug elimination. The concentration of drug in the circulation is given by

$$C = (D/V)e^{-k_{el}t} \tag{13.2}$$

The overall rate constant, k_{el}, controls the rate of drug loss. Similarly, cumulative urinary excretion of unchanged drug was described by

$$A_u = A_u^{\infty}(1 - e^{-k_{el}t}) \tag{13.3}$$

where $A_u^{\infty} = D(k_e/k_{el})$. This equation can be expressed in sigma-minus form as

$$\log(A_u^{\infty} - A_u) = \log A_u^{\infty} - (k_{el}/2.3)t \tag{13.4}$$

The overall elimination rate constant, k_{el}, controls the time dependency of urinary excretion, not k_e, which is the rate constant for urinary excretion.

The rate of change in the amount of metabolite in the body is given by

$$dM/dt = k_m A - k_{me}M \tag{13.5}$$

where M is the amount of metabolite in the body, k_{me} is the rate constant for metabolite loss, and k_m is the rate constant that controls the rate of metabolite formation. The value of A is given by Equation 13.1. Incorporating that expression into Equation 13.5 and integrating yields

$$M = \frac{A_0 k_m}{k_{me} - k_{el}}(e^{-k_{el}t} - e^{-k_{me}t}) \tag{13.6}$$

This equation describes the amount of metabolite in the body with respect to time. There are subtle differences between this equation and Equation 11.3, which describes the amount of drug in the body with first-order absorption and elimination. In that situation, only two rate constants, k_a and k_{el}, were involved. In this more complex situation, three constants, k_m, k_{me}, and k_{el}, are involved. The constant k_{el} reflects the loss of drug from the body by all processes. The rate constant for metabolite formation, k_m, plays a role in the overall scenario as a time-independent constant. Thus, the time course for the amount of metabolite in the body is controlled by the overall constant for loss of drug and the overall constant for loss of metabolite.

Analysis of Metabolite Concentrations in Plasma, and Urinary Excretion

In considering the time course of the amounts or concentrations of unchanged drug in the model with first-order absorption and elimination, three possible situations were established in which $k_a > k_{el}$, $k_a < k_{el}$, and $k_a = k_{el}$. The same situation frequently occurs with metabolites. That is, the overall rate constant for loss of drug, k_{el}, may be greater than, equal to, or less than the overall rate constant for elimination of metabolite, k_{me}.

The primary objective of drug metabolism is to produce a more water-soluble and, hence, more rapidly excretable derivative of the parent drug (1). Therefore, k_{me} would be expected to be greater than k_{el} in most cases. However, sometimes the metabolite has a longer intrinsic elimination half-life than the parent drug, and k_{el} is greater than k_{me}.

In Equation 13.6, for the case where k_{el} is greater than k_{me}, as time increases, the term $e^{-k_{el}t}$ will approach zero before the term $e^{-k_{me}t}$, and the equation will reduce to Equation 13.7, which rearranges to Equation 13.8 to keep the exponential term positive.

$$M = [A_0 k_m / (k_{me} - k_{el})] (-e^{-k_{me}t}) \qquad (13.7)$$

$$M = [A_0 k_m / (k_{el} - k_{me})] (e^{-k_{me}t}) \qquad (13.8)$$

Thus, the profile of the amount of metabolite in the body after an intravenous dose of parent drug can be interpreted as in Figure 13.1. The value k_{me} is obtained from

$$k_{me} = [\text{intercept} (k_{el} - k_{me})] / A_0 \qquad (13.9)$$

This method of interpretation is straightforward, but occurs only when $k_{el} > k_{me}$.

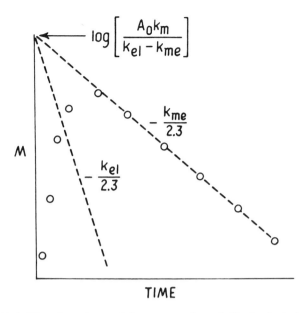

Figure 13.1. Time dependency of the amount of metabolite in the body following intravenous bolus injection of parent drug. The profile is interpreted in terms of Equation 13.6, with $k_{el} > k_{me}$.

The second situation, where the rate constant for metabolite elimination is greater than that for the parent drug, is described in Figure 13.2. In this case, $k_{me} > k_{el}$. As time increases, the term $e^{-k_{me}t}$ in Equation 13.6 will approach zero before the exponential term $e^{-k_{el}t}$; therefore, the equation will then reduce to

$$M = [A_0 k_m/(k_{me} - k_{el})] (e^{-k_{el}t}) \qquad (13.10)$$

This expression shows that the terminal linear portion of the metabolite profile in plasma is controlled by k_{el} (i.e., the rate constant for overall loss of drug from the body). In this case, the value of k_{me} is obtained from residuals, and the value of the common intercept of the terminal and residual slopes at time zero is $\log [A_0 k_m/(k_{me} - k_{el})]$. The value k_m is then obtained from

$$k_m = [\text{intercept } (k_{me} - k_{el})]/A_0 \qquad (13.11)$$

A number of factors can be learned by comparing the two situations represented by Figures 13.1 and 13.2. First, two possible ways to analyze metabolite data exist. Unless additional information is available, distin-

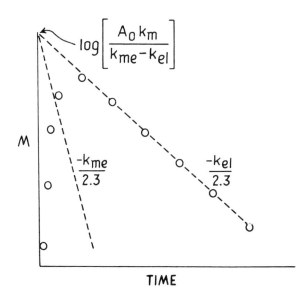

Figure 13.2. Time dependency of the amount of metabolite in the body following intravenous bolus injection of parent drug. The profile is interpreted in terms of Equation 13.6, with $k_{me} > k_{el}$.

guishing the correct from the incorrect method is impossible. That is, does the terminal linear slope of the metabolite profile represent k_{el} or k_{me}? This dilemma is similar to the flip-flop model that was discussed in Chapter 11. The additional information necessary to resolve this problem can be obtained from the elimination slope for unchanged drug. This plot will yield k_{el} directly, so that the two constants can then be distinguished from each other.

The second factor to be learned by comparing Figures 13.2 and 13.3 is that the observed terminal linear portion of the metabolite profile can have a slope that is less than that of the parent drug (when $k_{el} > k_{me}$), but it cannot have a slope that is greater than that of the parent drug. If k_{me} is greater than k_{el}, then the terminal slope of the metabolite profile is controlled by k_{el}. If the terminal slope for the metabolite appears to be steeper than that of the parent drug, then probably something is wrong with the assay.

Measurement of metabolites in urine is very common because metabolites frequently occur at much higher concentrations in urine than in the circulation. Appropriate expressions for urinary excretion of unchanged drug were given in Equation 10.28 and in sigma-minus form in Equation 10.30.

The analogous expressions for urinary metabolite data are based on the rate equation:

$$\frac{dM_u}{dt} = k_{me}M = \frac{k_{me}A_0k_m}{k_{me} - k_{el}} (e^{-k_{el}t} - e^{-k_{me}t}) \qquad (13.12)$$

where M_u is the amount of metabolite excreted in urine. This equation can be solved for M_u:

$$M_u = \frac{A_0k_m}{k_{el}} \left[1 - \frac{1}{k_{me} - k_{el}} (k_{me}e^{-k_{el}t} - k_{el}e^{-k_{me}t}) \right] \qquad (13.13)$$

Because the function $A_0(k_m/k_{el}) = M_u^\infty$, Equation 13.13 can be rewritten as

$$M_u = M_u^\infty \left[1 - \frac{1}{k_{me} - k_{el}} (k_{me}e^{-k_{el}t} - k_{el}e^{-k_{me}t}) \right] \qquad (13.14)$$

The time dependency of this equation can be examined in the same way as that of Equation 13.6. As in that equation, depending on the relative magnitude of k_{el} and k_{me}, one or the other of the two exponential terms in Equation 13.14 approaches zero with increasing time; therefore, during the terminal linear portion of the cumulative urinary excretion profile, Equation 13.14 may reduce to

$$M_u = M_u^\infty 1 - [1/(k_{me} - k_{el})] (-k_{el}e^{-k_{me}t}) \qquad (13.15)$$

and

$$M_u = M_u^\infty 1 - [1/(k_{me} - k_{el})] (k_{me}e^{-k_{el}t}) \qquad (13.16)$$

Expressed in sigma-minus form, these equations become, respectively, Equations 13.17 and 13.18.

$$\log (M_u^\infty - M_u) = \log \{M_u^\infty [k_{el}/(k_{el} - k_{me})]\} - (k_{me}/2.3)t \qquad (13.17)$$

$$\log (M_u^\infty - M_u) = \log \{M_u^\infty [k_{me}/(k_{me} - k_{el})]\} - (k_{el}/2.3)t \qquad (13.18)$$

These two equations present the same quandary as occurred with the plasma data, reflected in Equations 13.6, 13.8, and 13.10. If $\log (M_u^\infty - M_u)$ is plotted versus time, a plot is obtained that is at first curved, but then becomes linear as the contribution of either $e^{-k_{el}t}$ or $e^{-k_{me}t}$ in Equation 13.14 drops out, and the log-linear relationships described by Equations 13.17 or 13.18 are obtained. However, without additional information, determining which of these equations is appropriate is not possible.

Resolving the Pharmacokinetics of Metabolites and Parent Drugs

The problem of resolving the pharmacokinetics of metabolite and parent drug is best illustrated with a numerical example. Suppose 100 mg of a drug was administered by rapid bolus intravenous injection to a patient. Metabolite voided in urine is collected during a 50-h postdose period. The quantity of metabolite remaining to be excreted in urine, expressed in equivalents of unchanged drug, is given in Table 13.2. A plot of log $(M_u^\infty - M_u)$ versus time, would yield a curve similar to that shown in Figure 13.3.

Table 13.2—Quantity of Metabolite Recovered in Urine

Time (h)	Cumulative M_u (mg)	$M_u^\infty - M_u$ (mg)
0	0	80
0.5	1.1	78.9
1	3.1	76.9
2	10.5	69.5
5	35.3	44.7
10	62.2	17.8
15	73.4	6.6
20	77.5	2.5
25	79.1	0.9
30	79.7	0.3
40	80.0	0
50	80.0	0

NOTE: All values were obtained during a 50-h period following a single 100-mg bolus intravenous injection of parent drug.

These data can now be interpreted in two different ways depending on whether k_{el} or k_{me} is the larger rate constant. If k_{el} is larger, Equation 13.17 is appropriate; if k_{me} is larger, Equation 13.18 is appropriate. The calculations involved and the results obtained using these different approaches are shown in Table 13.3. The half-life of the terminal log-linear slope is 3.4 h. If Equation 13.17 is assumed, then $k_{me} = 0.693/3.4 = 0.2$ h^{-1}. If, on the other hand, Equation 13.18 is assumed, then this value is assigned to k_{el}. The intercept of the terminal portion of the log-linear curve on the ordinate at time zero is 140 mg. From this value and known values of k_{me} or k_{el}, k_{el} is calculated to be 0.47 h^{-1} from Equation 13.17, whereas k_{me} is calculated to have this value from Equation 13.18. Further substitutions yield values of 0.38 h^{-1} and 0.09 h^{-1} for k_m and k_e, respec-

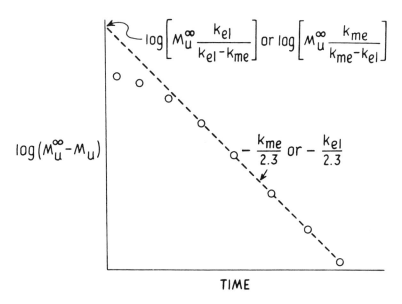

$$\log\left[M_u^\infty \frac{k_{el}}{k_{el}-k_{me}}\right] \text{ or } \log\left[M_u^\infty \frac{k_{me}}{k_{me}-k_{el}}\right]$$

$\log(M_u^\infty - M_u)$

$-\dfrac{k_{me}}{2.3}$ or $-\dfrac{k_{el}}{2.3}$

TIME

Figure 13.3. Plot of log $(M_u^\infty - M_u)$ versus time from data in Table 13.2. Interpretation is based on Equations 13.17 and 13.18.

tively, from Equation 13.17, and 0.16 h^{-1} and 0.04 h^{-1}, respectively, from Equation 13.18. Therefore, two completely different sets of parameter values are obtained depending on the assumption of the relative values of k_{el} and k_{me}.

Unless some additional data are available, determining which of these two sets of results is correct is impossible. However, this Gordian knot can be untied by two methods. The first method is to identify the value of k_{el} from the elimination slope of the plasma profile or urinary excretion data for the parent drug. If the terminal elimination rate constant for the metabolite is approximately equal to that of unchanged drug, then Equation 13.18 probably applies because k_{el} is most likely smaller than k_{me}. If, on the other hand, the terminal elimination rate constant for the metabolite is smaller than that for the unchanged drug, then Equation 13.17 applies because k_{me} is most likely smaller than k_{el}. Another approach is to dose the metabolite, if it is available, and thereby establish k_{me} independent of any influence from the parent drug.

It is evident from this brief treatment that pharmacokinetic characterization of metabolite formation and excretion is difficult. The example used here is based on formation of a single metabolite by a nonsaturable mechanism following intravenous dosing of a drug. In practice, the situation is more complex and more difficult to resolve. For example, the drug may be given orally so that the drug absorption constant must be taken into account. Drugs may form more than one metabolite, and one metabolite may be transformed to another in the body. Some metabolic pathways may be parallel, and some may be more saturable than others (2–4). For complete characterization of metabolite kinetics, having sufficient pure metabolite is desirable so that it can be dosed and its pharmacokinetics examined in the absence of other substances, particularly the parent drug (5,6).

Table 13.3—Pharmacokinetic Parameters

Equation 13.17	Equation 13.18
$t_{1/2} = 3.4$ h	$t_{1/2} = 3.4$ h
$k_{me} = 0.2$ h^{-1}	$k_{el} = 0.2$ h^{-1}
$M_u^\infty = 80$ mg	$M_u^\infty = 80$ mg
$M_u^\infty \left(\dfrac{k_{el}}{k_{el} - k_{me}} \right) = 140$ mg	$M_u^\tau \left(\dfrac{k_{me}}{k_{me} - k_{el}} \right) = 140$ mg
$\dfrac{k_{el}}{k_{el} - k_{me}} = \dfrac{140}{80} = 1.75$	$\dfrac{k_{me}}{k_{me} - k_{el}} = \dfrac{140}{80} = 1.75$
$k_{el} = 0.47$ h^{-1}	$k_{me} = 0.47$ h^{-1}
$k_m = \dfrac{k_{el} M_u^\infty}{D} = \dfrac{0.47 \times 80}{100} = 0.38$ h^{-1}	$k_m = \dfrac{k_{el} M_u^\infty}{D} = \dfrac{0.2 \times 80}{100} = 0.16$ h^{-1}
$k_e = k_{el} - k_m = 0.47 - 0.38 = 0.09$ h^{-1}	$k_e = k_{el} - k_m = 0.2 - 0.16 = 0.04$ h^{-1}

NOTE: All parameters are based on urinary excretion data from Table 13.2.

Summary

1. Metabolite formation and excretion can be described in terms of catenary chain kinetics.

2. The primary objective of drug metabolism is to generate more water-soluble and rapidly excreted compounds. However, in many instances the metabolite may be excreted at a slower rate than the parent drug.

3. Because of the close relationship between the kinetic behavior of parent drug and its metabolite(s), care must be exercised when parameter values are assigned when metabolite data are analyzed. This is particularly important when the rate for metabolite elimination is faster than the overall elimination rate for the parent drug.

Literature Cited

1. Taylor, J. A. Clin. Pharmacol. Ther., **1972**, 13, 710–718.
2. Levy, G. J. Pharm. Sci., **1965**, 54, 959–967.
3. Levy, G.; Vogel, A. W.; Amsel, L. P. J. Pharm Sci., **1969**, 58, 503–504.
4. Hewick, D. S.; McEwen, J. J. Pharm. Pharmacol., **1973**, 25, 458–465.
5. Tse, F. L. S; Welling, P. G. Biopharm. Drug Disp., **1980**, 1, 221–223.
6. Tse, F. L. S.; Welling, P. G. Res. Comm. Substance Abuse, **1980**, 1, 185–195.

Problems

1. A drug (100 mg) is dosed to a 70-kg male patient by rapid IV injection. The drug does not bind to plasma proteins, distributes into a volume equivalent to that of blood, and has a plasma clearance of 50 mL/min. The drug is cleared from the body as unchanged drug and as one metabolite. Both compounds are voided quantitatively into the urine. A sigma-minus plot of metabolite in urine data yielded a rate constant of 0.2 h^{-1} and total urinary excretion of metabolite accounted for 25% of the dose. Calculate the following: (i) $k_e(h^{-1})$, (ii) $k_m(h^{-1})$, and (iii) $k_{me}(h^{-1})$.

2. A drug (100 mg) is dosed orally to a patient. Only 20% of the dose is recovered in the feces. Of this, one-half is recovered as unchanged drug and may be assumed not to have been absorbed. Sixty percent of the original dose appears in urine as unchanged drug and the balance as urinary metabolites. A sigma-minus plot of urinary unchanged drug yielded an apparent elimination rate constant of 0.3 h^{-1}, and the intercept of the linear portion of the plot, extrapolated to time zero, was 75 mg. Calculate the following: (i) k_e, (ii) k_m, and (iii) the absorption rate constant k_a.

3. One-half of an intravenously dosed drug is voided unchanged in urine, and the balance of the drug is metabolized to inactive metabolites. The decline in plasma levels of unchanged drug is first-order and has a $t_{1/2}$ of 3 h. What is the value of the first-order rate constant obtained from a sigma-minus plot of unchanged drug in urine?

4. A drug, which gives rise to a single metabolite that is excreted in urine, has a biological half-life of 4 h. When the metabolite is administered alone, a biological half-life of 2 h results. What would the observed biological half-life of the metabolite be if measured following administration of parent drug?

5. What would the observed metabolite half-life in plasma be following administration of parent drug if the drug half-life was 4 h and the metabolite half-life, when administered alone, was 6 h?

14

The Two-Compartment Open Model with Intravenous or Oral Administration

The pharmacokinetic treatment in preceding chapters has been based on the one-compartment model. That is, the drug, after introduction into the body, is assumed to distribute rapidly into an apparently homogeneous volume.

Description of the Two-Compartment Model

For many drugs this simple approach is inadequate. The drug may not rapidly distribute into an apparently homogeneous volume, but may distribute more slowly into some tissues than others, and variable lengths of time may elapse before equilibrium is reached between drug concentrations, or amounts, in different body tissues and fluids. This situation is illustrated in Scheme 14.1. In the scheme, the central compartment represents plasma water and any other tissues or fluids into which the drug rapidly equilibrates. The other compartments in the scheme represent either single tissues or groups of tissues into which drug equilibrates at a slower rate than those of the central compartment. This model is very complex and cannot be characterized simply by measuring drug concentrations in plasma or urinary excretion. However, a less complex version of the model is obtained by combining all of the tissues outside of the central compartment and adding the separate rate constants. Scheme

0065-7719/86/0185-0213$08.00/1
© 1986 American Chemical Society

14.2, which is known as the two-compartment open model, is thus obtained. This particular version of the model represents the situation where drug is introduced into the central compartment (of which the blood, plasma, or serum are generally representative); distributes between the central compartment and the second, or peripheral compartment; and is eliminated from the central compartment (1–4).

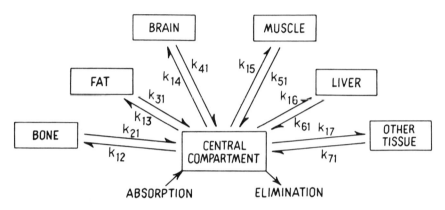

Scheme 14.1. Distribution of drug between the central compartment and various body tissues and fluids.

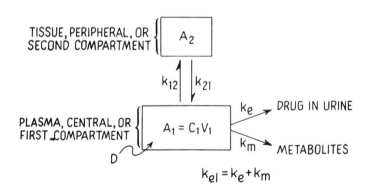

Scheme 14.2. The two-compartment open model with rapid intravenous injection.

Several variations of this model have been described. For example, drug could be introduced into, or could be eliminated from, the tissue and plasma compartments simultaneously, or drug could conceivably be eliminated exclusively from the second, or tissue, compartment (5). However, the model in Scheme 14.2 is the most common and makes good anatomical sense. Intravenous dosage always delivers drug directly into the plasma compartment. Similarly, drug elimination occurs principally via the liver or kidney, and these organs are intimately associated with, if not part of, the plasma compartment because of rapid blood flow through these organs and rapid equilibrium of substances between these organs and blood. Each compartment has three names. The plasma compartment is also called the central or first compartment. Similarly, the tissue compartment is also known as the peripheral or second compartment. These names are largely self-explanatory and are synonymous within each compartment. Some drugs that have been shown to obey two- or multicompartment model kinetics are shown in the list below.

Some Drugs That Have Been Shown to Obey Two- or Multicompartment Model Kinetics in the Body

Amphetamine	Methicillin
Chlordiazepoxide	Ouabain
Digoxin	Oxacillin
Digitoxin	Pentaerythritol
Ephedrine	Sulfamethazine
Ethchlorvynol	Sulfisoxazole
Gentamicin	Theophylline
Lidocaine	Warfarin

In the one-compartment model, drug equilibrated very rapidly into those fluids and tissues that constituted the distribution volume. Thus, a plot of drug concentration versus time following intravenous dosage yielded a simple monoexponential curve, and a plot of the logarithm of the drug concentration versus time yielded a straight line. With the two-compartment model, a distinctive curve is obtained that readily distinguishes the two-compartment model from the one-compartment model.

The sequence of events in the two-compartment model is as follows: After the drug is initially introduced into the first compartment by bolus intravenous injection, initial and rapid distribution into those fluids and tissues that constitute the first compartment occurs. At the same time, drug starts to disperse into the less accessible and more slowly equilibrating tissues and fluids that constitute the second compartment. Of course, drug is simultaneously eliminated from the first compartment. Because drug is not only being eliminated (excreted or metabolized) but is also being taken up by the second-compartment tissues and fluids during the early postdose period, rapid net loss of drug from the first compartment and a rapid decline in plasma concentrations occurs. This period of rapidly falling drug concentrations due to the combined effects of tissue uptake and elimination is called the α phase. After a certain period of time, dependent on the magnitude of the "microscopic" rate constants between the compartments, k_{12} and k_{21} in Scheme 14.2, drug will equilibrate between the various tissues and fluids, and net loss of drug from the first compartment due to distribution will no longer occur. Even though equilibrium is reached between the two compartments at the end of the α phase, the concentration of drug is not necessarily equal in the two compartments. The concentration of drug in tissue may be less or greater than that in the first compartment, but the concentrations will nonetheless be at equilibrium. Because the second compartment usually comprises several organs and tissues, the concentration of drug in this compartment is unlikely to be homogeneous.

Once equilibrium is reached between the two compartments, the rate of drug loss from the bloodstream is reduced. This period of more slowly declining blood levels is the β phase. The type of drug profile that occurs in this situation is shown in Figure 14.1, which shows the rapid decline of drug concentrations during the α phase, and the relatively slow decline during the β phase.

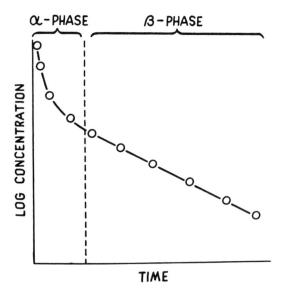

Figure 14.1. Blood levels of a drug that obeys two-compartment model kinetics following bolus intravenous injection.

Interpretation of Drug Concentration Profiles in Plasma To Obtain Parameter Estimates

Having established the kinetic model in Scheme 14.1, and having described the type of blood level curve that occurs in Figure 14.1, developing the appropriate equations that describe the drug profile profile in plasma is now necessary.

The rates of change in the amounts of drug in the first and second compartments, and also the cumulative amount of drug voided in urine with respect to time, are given by Equations 14.1 through 14.3.

$$dA_1/dt = k_{21}A_2 - (k_{12} + k_{el}) A_1 \tag{14.1}$$

$$dA_2/dt = k_{12}A_1 - k_{21}A_2 \tag{14.2}$$

$$dA_u/dt = k_e A_1 \tag{14.3}$$

These equations can be solved simultaneously to obtain

$$A_1 = [D/(\alpha - \beta)][(k_{21} - \beta)e^{-\beta t} - (k_{21} - \alpha)e^{-\alpha t}] \tag{14.4}$$

$$A_2 = [Dk_{12}/(\alpha - \beta)](e^{-\beta t} - e^{-\alpha t}) \tag{14.5}$$

$$A_u = A_u^{\infty}\left[1 - \frac{k_{el}}{(\alpha - \beta)}\left(\frac{k_{21} - \beta}{\beta}e^{-\beta t} - \frac{k_{21} - \alpha}{\alpha}e^{-\alpha t}\right)\right] \tag{14.6}$$

which represent the quantity of drug in the first compartment, the quantity of drug in the second compartment, and the quantity of drug cumulatively excreted unchanged in urine, respectively. The parameters α and β are complex rate constants that are related to the "microscopic" constants k_{12}, k_{21}, and k_{el} as shown in Equations 14.7 and 14.8.

$$\alpha = 0.5\{(k_{12} + k_{21} + k_{el}) + [(k_{12} + k_{21} + k_{el})^2 - 4k_{21}k_{el}]^{1/2}\} \tag{14.7}$$

$$\beta = 0.5\{(k_{12} + k_{21} + k_{el}) - [(k_{12} + k_{21} + k_{el})^2 - 4k_{21}k_{el}]^{1/2}\} \tag{14.8}$$

The only difference in the right sides of these two equations is the sign separating the parenthetical term and the root function. These equations appear complex, but careful examination will show that the combined Equations 14.7 and 14.8 can be written

$$X = \frac{-b \pm \sqrt{b^2 - 4ac}}{2a} \tag{14.9}$$

This equation represents the two possible values of X in the quadratic equation:

$$aX^2 + bX + c = 0 \tag{14.10}$$

Equation 14.9 thus represents the two possible roots of Equation 14.10.

In exactly the same way, the values α and β are the two possible roots of a quadratic function that one obtains when obtaining simultaneous solutions for the rate Equations 14.1, 14.2, and 14.3.

The values α and β are therefore intimately related to the values of k_{12}, k_{21}, and k_{el}, and both α and β are influenced by all three rate constants. If k_{12} is very fast, then drug will distribute rapidly into peripheral tissue. Detecting a distribution phase in this case will be difficult, and the drug will tend to exhibit simple one-compartment model kinetics. The slower k_{12} becomes relative to the other microscopic constants, the slower the distribution phase, and the more two-compartment character is evident in the drug profile in plasma.

Examining the relationships between the values of α and β and the magnitude of the elimination rate constant, k_{el}, is interesting. For example if values of k_{12} and k_{21} were held constant, and the value of the elimination rate constant was varied over a fairly wide range, then for very high values of k_{el}, with very fast intrinsic elimination, the value of α would approach k_{el}. For very low values of k_{el} relative to the other microscopic constants, α approaches the sum of k_{12} and k_{21}. Because of the negative sign in Equation 14.8, the value of β is affected differently by changes in k_{el}. For instance, at high values of k_{el}, when elimination is rapid relative to k_{12} and k_{21}, the value of β approaches k_{21}. At very low values of k_{el}, β approaches zero.

The next task is to obtain estimates of the rate constants and other parameters associated with the model from the drug profile in plasma. Equation 14.4 can be rewritten in concentration form as

$$C = \frac{D}{V_1(\alpha - \beta)} [(k_{21} - \beta)e^{-\beta t} - (k_{21} - \alpha)e^{-\alpha t}] \qquad (14.11)$$

where V_1 is the volume of the first compartment. Equation 14.11 can be expressed in shorthand notation as

$$C = Ae^{-\alpha t} + Be^{-\beta t} \qquad (14.12)$$

In this equation, the values A and B relate to the parameters in Equation 14.4, as shown in Equations 14.13 and 14.14.

$$A = [D(k_{21} - \alpha)]/[V_1(\alpha - \beta)] \qquad (14.13)$$

$$B = [D(k_{21} - \beta)]/[V_1(\alpha - \beta)] \qquad (14.14)$$

Graphical Estimation of Kinetic Parameters

To obtain graphical estimates of the pharmacokinetic parameters associated with this model, plotting drug concentration data, as shown in

Figure 14.1, and stripping the curve to obtain estimates of the four constants, A, B, α, and β in Equation 14.12 is convenient. This procedure is demonstrated in Figure 14.2. According to Equations 14.7 and 14.8 the rate constant α must be greater than β; therefore, as time increases after dosing, the term $Ae^{-\alpha t}$ will approach zero before the term $Be^{-\beta t}$, and Equation 14.12 will reduce to

$$C = Be^{-\beta t}, \quad \text{or} \quad \log C = \log B - (\beta/2.3)t \qquad (14.15)$$

The swiftly declining portion of the drug profile is the α phase. The portion in which only Equation 14.15 contributes to the curve, the more slowly declining portion, is the β phase.

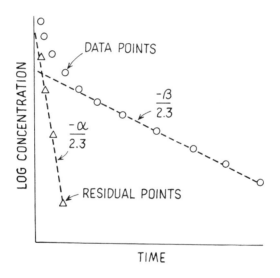

Figure 14.2. Method to obtain initial estimates of the constants A, B, α, and β in equation 14.12 from the blood profile of a drug that obeys two-compartment model kinetics after bolus intravenous injection.

The value β is thus obtained from the terminal linear portion of the log concentration versus time curve, and the intercept of this linear portion extrapolated back to time zero is the concentration term B. The values of A and α are obtained by the method of residuals or curve stripping, described in Chapter 11 for the one-compartment model with first-order absorption. In this case, however, residual values are obtained by subtracting the values on the extrapolated portion of the β slope from the actual data values obtained during the α phase. The residual values thus obtained are plotted as shown in Figure 14.2. The slope of the residual line gives the value of α and the intercept at time zero gives the value A. Proof that the slope and intercepts of the residual line represent α and A is given by

$$R = Ae^{-\alpha t} + Be^{-\beta t} - Be^{-\beta t} \tag{14.16}$$

in which the right side of Equation 14.15 is subtracted from the right side of Equation 14.12. The logarithmic form of the resulting residual function is given by

$$\log R = \log A - (\alpha/2.3)\, t \tag{14.17}$$

Numerical values have thus been obtained for the concentration terms A and B and the rate constants α and β. Using these terms to find numerical values for the microscopic constants and other values associated with the model in Scheme 14.2 is a simple process.

The first relationship to note is that the initial drug concentration at time zero, C_0, which is the concentration obtained when the drug has distributed within the first compartment but has not yet started to enter the second compartment, is equal to $A + B$, as in

$$C_0 = A + B \tag{14.18}$$

As $C_0 = D/V_1$, Equation 14.18 can be rewritten as

$$D/V_1 = A + B \tag{14.19}$$

which rearranges to give the value V_1 in terms of the dose and two intercepts, as in

$$V_1 = D/(A + B) \tag{14.20}$$

Estimates for the rate constants k_{12}, k_{21}, and k_{el} are obtained in a sequential manner, by solving for one, and then using that value to solve for the next. The first constant to solve for is k_{21}, by means of Equation 14.13, which is rearranged for convenience as

$$k_{21} - \alpha = AV_1(\beta - \alpha)/D \tag{14.21}$$

Equation 14.21 rearranges further to

$$k_{21} = \alpha + AV_1(\beta - \alpha)/D \tag{14.22}$$

Equation 14.20 can be substituted into Equation 14.22, which then rearranges to Equation 14.23.

$$k_{21} = (A\beta + B\alpha)/(A + B) \qquad (14.23)$$

In this equation, the unknown constant, k_{21}, is expressed in terms of four known values: A, α, B, and β.

The next constant to solve for is k_{el} by using the relationships in Equations 14.7 and 14.8. If α is multiplied by β, then similar multiplication of the right side of Equations 14.7 and 14.8 and appropriate cancellation of like terms yields the simple relationship

$$\alpha\beta = k_{21}k_{el} \qquad (14.24)$$

Equation 14.24 rearranges to

$$k_{el} = \alpha\beta/k_{21} \qquad (14.25)$$

which describes k_{el} in terms of known values. The known values on the right side of Equation 14.25 include the microscopic constant k_{21}.

The third microscopic constant k_{12} is obtained by adding α and β in terms of the relationships in Equations 14.7 and 14.8. Addition of these equations yields Equation 14.26, which rearranges to Equation 14.27.

$$\alpha + \beta = k_{12} + k_{21} + k_{el} \qquad (14.26)$$

$$k_{12} = \alpha + \beta - k_{21} - k_{el} \qquad (14.27)$$

Recognizing the difference between k_{el} and β is important. From the model in Scheme 14.2, k_{el} is the intrinsic rate constant for loss of drug from the body, or more accurately, from the first compartment. However, the actual elimination slope obtained from drug concentration data is given by β, and the overall drug elimination half-life, or biological half-life, is given by

$$t_{1/2(\beta)} = 0.693/\beta \qquad (14.28)$$

In exactly the same way, the half-life of α, or the fast disposition phase of the drug profile, is given by

$$t_{1/2(\alpha)} = 0.693/\alpha \qquad (14.29)$$

Derivation of AUC$^{0\to\infty}$, Plasma Clearance, and Renal Clearance

The area under the drug-plasma curve in this model can be calculated by means of the trapezoidal rule in the same way as in the one-compartment model because the area is a model-independent parameter. In the present model, the "end correction" that may be necessary to convert a truncated area to an area to infinite time is given by

$$\text{end correction} = C_t/\beta \tag{14.30}$$

The area under the curve from zero to infinite time can be expressed in pharmacokinetic terms by integrating Equation 14.11 or 14.12 between the limits of zero and infinite time. Integration of Equation 14.11 yields Equation 14.31, and similar integration of Equation 14.12 yields Equation 14.32.

$$\text{AUC}^{0\to\infty} = (A/\alpha) + (B/\beta) \tag{14.31}$$

$$\text{AUC}^{0\to\infty} = D/(V_1 k_{el}) \tag{14.32}$$

Proving that Equations 14.31 and 14.32 are identical is an interesting exercise.

From the one-compartment model discussion, plasma clearance is known to be equal to the intravenous dose divided by the area under the drug concentration curve from zero to infinite time. The same situation occurs with the two-compartment model. As two possible expressions have been written for the area under the curve, Equations 14.31 and 14.32, two expressions can also be written for plasma clearance. Equation 14.31 yields Equation 14.33, and Equation 14.32 yields Equation 14.34.

$$Cl_p = D/[(A/\alpha) + (B/\beta)] \tag{14.33}$$

$$Cl_p = D/(D/V_1 k_{el}) = V_1 k_{el} \tag{14.34}$$

The expression $V_1 k_{el}$ in Equation 14.34 is similar to the clearance expression $V k_{el}$ in the one-compartment case. The renal clearance is readily obtained by dividing the total quantity of drug recovered in urine by the area under the plasma curve, or alternatively by multiplying the plasma clearance by the ratio k_e/k_{el}, as in Equation 14.35.

$$Cl_r = \frac{A_u^\infty}{(A/\alpha)(B/\beta)} = V_1 k_{el}\left(\frac{k_e}{k_{el}}\right) = V_1 k_e \tag{14.35}$$

Volume of Distribution at Equilibrium

Just as the term V is used to represent the overall distribution volume of a drug that obeys one-compartment model kinetics, so the term V_{dss} is used to describe the volume that a drug obeying two-compartment model kinetics would occupy if the distribution volume at equilibrium were homogeneous. The overall drug distribution volume is derived in the following way. At steady state, the clearance of drug between the first and second compartments of the two-compartment model should be equal:

$$V_1 k_{12} = V_2 k_{21} \tag{14.36}$$

which rearranges to

$$V_2 = V_1 k_{12}/k_{21} \tag{14.37}$$

Because V_{dss}, or the total distribution volume, is equal to $V_1 + V_2$, the distribution volume can be described in terms of V_1 and the microscopic constants k_{12} and k_{el}, as in Equation 14.38.

$$V_{dss} = V_1 + V_1(k_{12}/k_{21}) = V_1[1 + (k_{12}/k_{21})] \tag{14.38}$$

This expression is used most often to describe the overall drug distribution volume with the two-compartment model.

Other methods have been used to describe the overall distribution volume of a drug that obeys two-compartment model kinetics. The two methods that are most commonly used lead to the overall distribution volumes $V_{d(extrap)}$ and $V_{d\beta}$. The second of these, $V_{d\beta}$, is also known as $V_{d(area)}$ (6).

The term $V_{d(extrap)}$ is derived from the assumption that drug is homogeneously distributed in the body during the β phase of the drug profile. If the β phase is then extrapolated back to time zero to obtain point B as in Figure 14.2, then an estimate of the drug concentration in the equilibrium condition before any drug loss from the body should be provided:

$$V_{d(extrap)} = D/B \tag{14.39}$$

From Equation 14.14, B is related to the dose, V_1, and various rate constants as in

$$B = [D(k_{21} - \beta)]/[V_1 (\alpha - \beta)] \tag{14.40}$$

As the volume term $V_{d(extrap)}$ is equal to the dose divided by the intercept B (Equation 14.39), Equation 14.40 can be substituted into Equation 14.39 to obtain the new equation:

$$V_{d(extrap)} = [V_1(\alpha - \beta)]/[(k_{21} - \beta)] \qquad (14.41)$$

This equation is the standard form of the relationship among $V_{d(extrap)}$, V_1, and rate constants associated with the two-compartment model.

The term $V_{d\beta}$, or $V_{d(area)}$, is derived from the relationship:

$$AUC^{0 \to \infty} = D/(V_{d\beta}\beta) \qquad (14.42)$$

This equation is analogous to

$$AUC^{0 \to \infty} = D/(Vk_{el}) \qquad (14.43)$$

that was used to relate area, dose, and plasma clearance for the one-compartment model in Chapter 10. In Equation 14.42 the denominator $V_{d\beta}\beta$ is the plasma clearance. Another expression for plasma clearance with the two-compartment model is V_1k_{el}, as in

$$\text{plasma clearance} = V_1k_{el} \qquad (14.44)$$

Equating the two different terms for plasma clearance for the two-compartment model is shown by

$$V_1k_{el} = V_{d\beta}\beta \qquad (14.45)$$

which rearranges to

$$V_{d\beta} = V_1(k_{el}/\beta) \qquad (14.46)$$

which gives the overall volume term, $V_{d\beta}$, or $V_{d(area)}$, in terms of V_1, k_{el}, and β. Because $\alpha\beta = k_{21}k_{el}$, Equation 14.46 can be written in the alternative form:

$$V_{d\beta} = V_1(\alpha/k_{21}) \qquad (14.47)$$

Thus, three expressions have been derived to describe the overall drug distribution volume at equilibrium, V_{dss}, $V_{d(extrap)}$, and $V_{d\beta}$. Note that the term V_{dss} does not contain an elimination rate constant in the form of β or k_{el}, but is dependent only on the distribution constants k_{12}, k_{21}, and V_1. The other volume terms are dependent on k_{el} or β and are thus elimination rate constant-dependent. To illustrate the dependency of

$V_{d(\text{extrap})}$ and $V_{d\beta}$ on drug elimination rate, consider the relationship between these values and the elimination rate-independent volume V_{dss} as k_{el} decreases in value. This relationship is illustrated in Equations 14.48 and 14.49.

$$V_{d(\text{extrap})} = \frac{V_1(\alpha - \beta)}{(k_{21} - \beta)} \overset{(\beta \to 0)}{=} V_1 \frac{\alpha}{k_{21}} = V_1 \frac{k_{12} + k_{21}}{k_{21}} = V_1 \left(1 + \frac{k_{12}}{k_{21}}\right) \quad (14.48)$$

$$V_{d\beta} = V_1 \frac{\alpha}{k_{21}} \overset{(k_{el} \to 0)}{=} V_1 \frac{k_{12} + k_{21}}{k_{21}} = V_1 \left(1 + \frac{k_{12}}{k_{21}}\right) \quad (14.49)$$

As k_{el} or β approach zero (and recall that if $k_{el} = 0$ then β must also equal zero) so the terms $V_{d(\text{extrap})}$ and $V_{d\beta}$ approach the value of V_{dss}. Both $V_{d(\text{extrap})}$ and $V_{d\beta}$, although used extensively in the literature, overestimate the overall distribution volume relative to the value V_{dss}. The degree of overestimation depends on how fast the drug is eliminated relative to the values of the distribution constants k_{12} and k_{21} (7).

The Kinetics of Tissue Distribution

For drugs that obey two-compartment model kinetics after intravenous administration, drug concentrations in blood, plasma, or serum decline initially at a fast rate because of combined tissue uptake and elimination, and decline subsequently at a slower rate.

While the drug is drawn out of plasma during the α distribution phase, it accumulates in tissue so that, as the amount of drug in plasma decreases, the amount of drug in tissue increases. This process continues until equilibrium is reached between the plasma and tissue compartments. The time at which equilibrium is achieved will mark the end of the α phase. Then, during the β phase, drug levels in both compartments will decline at the same rate, although the amount of drug in the two compartments may be different depending on the relative affinity of drug for various central and peripheral tissues. This situation is illustrated in Figure 14.3. The quantity of drug in the second compartment is represented as being greater than that in the first compartment during the β phase, but this is not necessarily the case.

The quantities of drug in the two compartments were described previously by Equations 14.4 and 14.5. Although the two equations are obviously different, they have identical time dependencies containing the rate constants α and β so that the rate of drug increase in tissue during the α phase following intravenous dosage will be the mirror image of the rate of decline in drug concentrations in plasma. During the β phase, drug levels in tissue and plasma will decline at the same rate according to the first-order rate constant β. During the α phase, the relative amounts

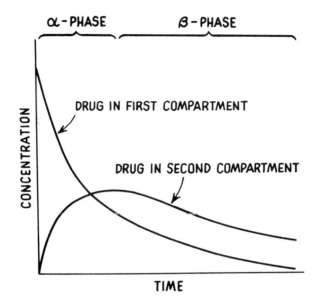

Figure 14.3. Drug concentrations in the first and second compartments of the two-compartment open model following bolus intravenous injection into the central compartment.

of drug in the two compartments are changing rapidly with respect to each other. However, during the β phase an equilibrium situation exists and the ratio of the quantity of drug in tissue to the quantity of drug in plasma should be constant.

This ratio can be established from the β phase segments of Equations 14.4 and 14.5. During the β phase of a drug profile in tissue or plasma the term $e^{-\alpha t}$ has reduced to zero so that Equations 14.4 and 14.5 collapse to Equations 14.50 and 14.51, respectively.

$$A_1 = [Dk_{12}/(\alpha - \beta)](k_{21} - \beta) e^{-\beta t} \tag{14.50}$$

$$A_2 = [Dk_{12}/(\alpha - \beta)] e^{-\beta t} \tag{14.51}$$

Dividing Equation 14.51 by Equation 14.50 and canceling like terms yields Equation 14.52.

$$A_2/A_1 = k_{12}/(k_{21} - \beta) = T/P \tag{14.52}$$

This equation indicates that the ratio of drug in tissue to drug in plasma, the T/P ratio, is given by k_{12} divided by the difference between k_{21} and β (i.e., the equilibrium ratio of drug in the two compartments is a function not only of the relative magnitude of the two rate constants, k_{12} and k_{21}, but also of the magnitude of β). Imagine the situation where k_{12} and k_{21} are both 0.1 h^{-1} and β is only 0.01 h^{-1}. The T/P ratio will then be 0.1/0.09 = 1.1. However, if β is 0.05 h^{-1}, then the T/P ratio will be 0.1/0.05 = 2.0. If β were 0.08 h^{-1}, then T/P = 0.1/0.02 = 5.0. Thus the ratio of the quantity of drug in tissue to that in the plasma compartment is influenced by the overall drug elimination rate.

The dependency of T/P on the drug elimination rate is similar to the elimination rate dependency of $V_{d(extrap)}$ and $V_{d\beta}$ described previously. Failure to recognize this dependency can lead to false conclusions regarding the influence (or lack of influence) of drug elimination on drug disposition in the body.

The equation for cumulative urinary excretion of drug with this model was given as Equation 14.6.

Obtaining Parameter Estimates from Urinary Excretion Data

Obtaining good estimates of pharmacokinetic parameters from urinary data with this model is difficult because of the model complexity and the difficulty of obtaining sufficiently frequent urine samples, even with water loading. However, given that satisfactory urine collection can be obtained, one way to analyze urinary excretion data is to construct sigma-minus plots in the same way as described previously for the one-compartment model (Chapter 11). During the postdistributive phase, that is, when the value of $e^{-\alpha t}$ approaches zero, Equation 14.6 reduces to

$$A_u = A_u^{\infty}\{1 - [k_{el}/(\alpha - \beta)][(k_{21} - \beta)/\beta]e^{-\beta t}\} \tag{14.53}$$

Because $\alpha\beta = k_{21}k_{el}$, Equation 14.53 can be rearranged to Equation 14.54.

$$\log (A_u^{\infty} - A_u) = \log \{A_u^{\infty}[k_{el}(k_{21} - \beta)/\beta(\alpha - \beta)]\} - (\beta/2.3)t \tag{14.54}$$

$$\log (A_u^{\infty} - A_u) = \log \{A_u^{\infty}[(\alpha - k_{el})/(\alpha - \beta)]\} - (\beta/2.3)t \tag{14.55}$$

This equation shows that if the logarithm of the amount of drug remaining to be excreted, $\log [A_u^{\infty} - A_u]$, is plotted against time, the situation illustrated in Figure 14.4 is obtained. The terminal linear portion of the plot is described by Equation 14.55. The rate constant β is obtained from the slope of the line and $\log [A_u(\alpha - k_{el})/(\alpha - \beta)]$ from the intercept at zero time. If residuals are taken in the same way as with the drug profile in plasma (i.e., by subtracting values on the extrapolated β slope from the actual values at early sampling times), a residual slope can be constructed that will have a slope of $-\alpha/2.3$ and an intercept of $\log \{A_u^{\infty}[1 - (\alpha - k_{el})/(\alpha - \beta)]\}$.

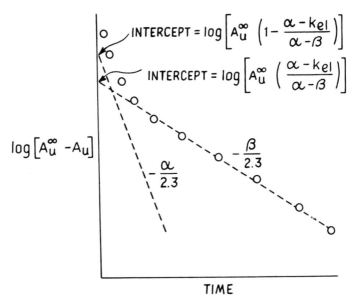

$$\text{INTERCEPT} = \log\left[A_u^\infty\left(1 - \frac{\alpha - k_{el}}{\alpha - \beta}\right)\right]$$

$$\text{INTERCEPT} = \log\left[A_u^\infty\left(\frac{\alpha - k_{el}}{\alpha - \beta}\right)\right]$$

$\log\left[A_u^\infty - A_u\right]$

$-\dfrac{\alpha}{2.3}$

$-\dfrac{\beta}{2.3}$

TIME

Figure 14.4. Plot of the logarithm of the amount of drug remaining to be excreted in urine versus time. Method of obtaining graphical estimates of pharmacokinetic parameters.

Knowing the values of the slopes and intercepts of the two lines, k_{el} can be solved as in Equation 14.56.

$$k_{el} = \alpha - [\text{intercept } (\alpha - \beta)/A_u^x] \tag{14.56}$$

After k_{el} is obtained, k_{21} can be obtained from Equation 14.57, and k_{12} from Equation 14.58.

$$k_{21} = \alpha\beta/k_{el} \tag{14.57}$$

$$k_{12} = \alpha + \beta - k_{el} - k_{21} \tag{14.58}$$

No volume calculations can be done with these data because urinary excretion of drug provides no information regarding concentrations of drug within the body compartments.

Although the preceding calculations are straightforward on a purely theoretical basis, good data are required for correct and accurate parameter estimation (i.e., accurate, frequent, and complete urine collections, and also accurate and specific assays). Accurate and specific assays are particularly important in urine analysis compared to plasma analysis because of the greater possibility of metabolite interference.

The Two-Compartment Model with First-Order Drug Input

The two-compartment model with first-order drug input is presented in Scheme 14.3, and a typical blood profile is shown in Figure 14.5. This model is similar to the model for the bolus intravenous case, except that a first-order absorption rate constant is included.

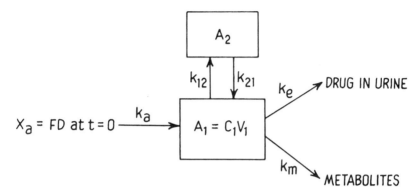

Scheme 14.3. Two-compartment open model with first-order drug input.

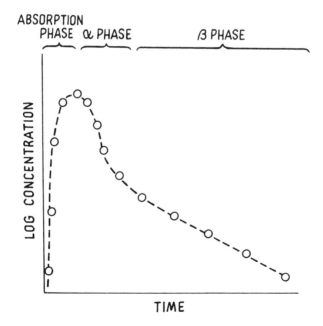

Figure 14.5. Blood concentration versus time profile of a drug that obeys two-compartment model kinetics following first-order drug input.

In this model, drug is assumed to be absorbed from the absorption site at a first-order rate. During the absorption phase and also extending beyond that phase, the drug distributes from the blood or plasma and all other fluids asociated with the first compartment into the less accessible, slowly equilibrating peripheral tissues that constitute the second compartment. When equilibrium is established then, as in the intravenous case, drug levels in the circulation and in tissue decline at a first-order rate controlled by the rate constant β. As shown in the figure, the three phases of the blood profile can be described as the absorption, α, and β phases.

Before describing the mathematics and methods of obtaining parameter values from this model, some words of caution are appropriate. This model contains many traps for the unwary, and analysis must be done with cognizance that several different methods can be used to analyze the data and to assign kinetic parameter values.

Detecting two- or multicompartment model kinetics following an oral dose of a drug is difficult, although such models may be evident after intravenous dosing. This difficulty is due to the absorption and α phases being of similar duration; therefore, the α, or distribution phase, will be obscured by the absorption phase. This condition not only prevents two-compartment model analysis but also throws further doubt on the significance of the absorption rate constant, k_a. A high probability of a flip-flop model occurrence also exists, not only between the absorption and elimination rate constants as discussed earlier for the one-compartment model (Chapter 11), but also between the k_a and α rate constants. Thus, incorrect values could be assigned to these two constants. Finally, because of the increased complexity of this model, more data points are required for accurate parameter characterization. Assigning numerical values to the various rate constants associated with the model is unrealistic unless sufficient data points exist to define each of the three phases of the drug profile (8,9).

From Scheme 14.3, the rates of change in the amounts of drug in the first and second compartments, and also the cumulative amount of drug voided in urine with respect to time, are given by Equations 14.59 through 14.61.

$$dA_1/dt = k_a X_a + k_{21}A_2 - (k_{12} + k_{el}) A_1 \qquad (14.59)$$

$$dA_2/dt = k_{12}A_1 - k_{21}A_2 \qquad (14.60)$$

$$dA_u/dt = k_e A_1 \qquad (14.61)$$

These equations can be solved simultaneously to obtain Equations 14.62 through 14.64.

$A_1 = FDk_a$

$$\times \left[\frac{(k_{21} - \alpha)}{(k_a - \alpha)(\beta - \alpha)} e^{-\alpha t} + \frac{(k_{21} - \beta)}{(k_a - \beta)(\alpha - \beta)} e^{-\beta t} \right.$$

$$\left. + \frac{(k_{21} - k_a)}{(\alpha - k_a)(\beta - k_a)} e^{-k_a t} \right]$$

$$(14.62)$$

$A_2 = FDk_a k_{21}$

$$\times \left[\frac{e^{-\alpha t}}{(k_a - \alpha)(\beta - \alpha)} + \frac{e^{-\beta t}}{(k_a - \beta)(\alpha - \beta)} + \frac{e^{-k_a t}}{(\alpha - k_a)(\beta - k_a)} \right] \quad (14.63)$$

$$A_u = A_u^{\infty} \left\{ 1 - k_a k_{el} \left[\frac{(k_{21} - \alpha)}{\alpha(k_a - \alpha)(\beta - \alpha)} e^{-\alpha t} + \frac{k_{21} - \beta}{\beta(\alpha - \beta)(k_a - \beta)} e^{-\beta t} \right.\right.$$

$$\left.\left. + \frac{(k_{12} - k_a)}{k_a(\alpha - k_a)(\beta - k_a)} e^{-k_a t} \right] \right\} \quad (14.64)$$

which represent the quantity of drug in the first compartment, the quantity of drug in the second compartment, and drug cumulatively excreted unchanged in the urine, respectively (10). In these equations, the constants α and β have identical relationships to k_{12}, k_{21}, and k_{el} that were established in the intravenous case (Equations 14.7 and 14.8). Equation 14.62, the amount of drug in the first compartment, can be rewritten in concentration form:

$$C = \frac{FDk_a}{V_1}$$

$$\times \left[\frac{(k_{21} - \alpha)}{(k_a - \alpha)(\beta - \alpha)} e^{-\alpha t} + \frac{(k_{21} - \beta)}{(k_a - \beta)(\alpha - \beta)} e^{-\beta t} \right.$$

$$\left. + \frac{(k_{21} - k_a)}{(\alpha - k_a)(\beta - k_a)} e^{-k_a t} \right]$$

$$(14.65)$$

Equations 14.62–14.65 are very similar. All of these expressions have the same time relationships, and they all contain the same three exponential functions, k_a, α, and β.

Drug Concentration in the First Compartment

In the intravenous case, the equation for C, Equation 14.11, was written in shorthand notation as Equation 14.12. Equation 14.65 can similarly be written in the form of

$$C = Ae^{-\alpha t} + Be^{-\beta t} + C'e^{-k_a t} \quad (14.66)$$

The symbol C' is used for the third concentration constant to differentiate it from the concentration in plasma term C. The three constants, A, B, and C', represent the groups of kinetic parameters in Equation 14.65 as shown in Equations 14.67, 14.68, and 14.69, respectively.

$$A = \frac{FDk_a(k_{21} - \alpha)}{V_1(k_a - \alpha)(\beta - \alpha)} \tag{14.67}$$

$$B = \frac{FDk_a(k_{21} - \beta)}{V_1(k_a - \beta)(\alpha - \beta)} \tag{14.68}$$

$$C' = \frac{FDk_a(k_{21} - k_a)}{V_1(\alpha - k_a)(\beta - k_a)} \tag{14.69}$$

The task at hand is to take a set of drug concentration versus time data and use it to obtain graphical estimates of all of the pharmacokinetic parameters associated with this model. Consider the drug concentration data in Table 14.1. The three sequential steps in the analysis of the data are shown in Figure 14.6.

The procedure is as follows. The data are first plotted on semilog-arithmic graph paper, and the terminal linear slope is assigned the value $-\beta/2.3$, and the extrapolated intercept at zero time is B. The first residual is then obtained by subtracting the values on the extrapolated portion of the β line from the actual data points during the pre-β portion of the curve. In this case, four data points were used to construct the β slope (because those points were on a straight line), leaving 10 data points including zero time to form the first residual. In the table, the first residual column is designated $C - \hat{C}$. The first residual has both negative and positive values depending on whether the data points fall above or below the extrapolated β line, as shown in Figure 14.6a. The positive values obtained from the first residual are then plotted on semilogarithmic graph paper, and the terminal linear descending portion of that curve is shown in Figure 14.6b. The last three residual points are linear, and a line is therefore constructed through these points and extrapolated back to time zero as in Figure 14.6b. This slope gives the rate constant α (assuming that $\alpha < k_a$) and the intercept is A.

To obtain the remaining two parameters, C' and k_a, the values on the extrapolated slope of the terminal portion of the first residual curve are subtracted from the values on the early nonlinear portion of the first residual curve to obtain the second residual. This procedure is described in Table 14.1 and shown in Figure 14.6b. In the table, the extrapolated first residual line is depicted as $\hat{C}$. The slope of the second residual, $C - \hat{C}$, is composed entirely of negative values reflecting the opposite direc-tion of this phase of the drug profile to that of the α and β phases, and

Table 14.1—Drug Concentration Data Analysis by the Method of Residuals

Time	Concentration (C)	First Residual		$\hat{C} = (C - \hat{C})$	Second Residual	
		$\hat{C}(27.1e^{-0.6t})$	$C - \hat{C}(residual)$		$C(116e^{-1.33t})$	$C - \hat{C}$
0.0	0.0	27.10	− 27.10	− 27.10	116.0	− 143.1
0.1	24.53	26.94	− 2.41	− 2.41	101.55	− 103.96
0.2	40.51	26.78	+ 13.73	13.73	88.91	− 75.18[a]
0.5	58.49	26.30	+ 32.19	32.19	59.66	− 27.47
1.0	52.28	25.52	+ 26.76	26.76	30.70	− 3.94
1.5	41.07	24.77	+ 16.30	16.30	15.78	
2.0	32.73	24.04	+ 8.69	8.69	8.11	
3.0	25.02	22.63	+ 2.39[b]			
4.0	21.95	21.32	+ 0.63			
6.0	18.95	18.91	+ 0.04			
8.0	16.77					
10.0	14.87[c]					
20.0	8.16					
40.0	2.46					

NOTE: Drug concentration in plasma data were obtained during a 40-h period for a drug that obeys the two-compartment kinetics with first-order absorption and elimination.
[a] Linear k_a phase, Intercept (C) = 143, $t_{\frac{1}{2}}$ = 0.23, and k_a = 3.01.
[b] Linear α phase, Intercept (A) = 116.0, $t_{\frac{1}{2}}$ = 0.52, and α = 1.33.
[c] Linear β phase, Intercept (B) = 27.1, $t_{\frac{1}{2}}$ = 11.5, and β = 0.06.

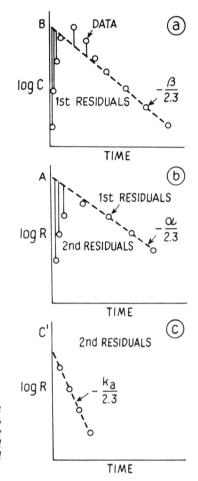

Figure 14.6. Method to obtain residuals from drug profile in Figure 14.5. (a) Terminal β slope and first residual obtained from Figure 14.5, (b) slope of first residual and method to obtain second residual, (c) slope of second residual.

also the negative value of the intercept of the second residual slope at zero time. To obtain the values of C' and k_a, the absolute values of the residuals in Table 14.1 are plotted, as shown in Figure 14.6c. These values should yield a straight line because this final slope is monoexponential, the α and β components now having been removed. The line has a slope of $-k_a/2.3$, and an intercept of C'.

The numerical values obtained from the data in Table 14.1 are summarized in

$$C = 116e^{-1.33t} + 27e^{-0.06t} - 143e^{-3.01t} \qquad (14.70)$$

The value C' is negative because of the negative values of the second residual slope in the table. Two good tests of whether the analysis is accurate are (i) to make sure that α, β, and k_a have different values from one another and increase in the order $\beta < \alpha < k_a$ (assuming no flip-flop situation), and (ii) to verify that concentration of drug in the bloodstream should be zero at zero time because no drug has been absorbed. When $t = 0$ in Equation 14.66, Equation 14.71 is obtained.

$$C = A + B + C' \tag{14.71}$$

Therefore, if the three constants A, B, and C' are added (C' is negative), a value should be obtained that equals or approaches zero.

The three concentration terms and three rate constants in Equation 14.70 can now be used to obtain values of the microscopic constants, k_{12}, k_{21}, and k_{el}. These calculations are done with Equations 14.67, 14.68, and 14.69, but removing the term k_a from the right side of these equations is convenient at first. To do this, each equation is divided by k_a to obtain the new functions P, Q, and R as in Equations 14.72, 14.73, and 14.74.

$$P = \frac{A}{k_a} = \frac{FD}{V_1}\left[\frac{(k_{21} - \alpha)}{(k_a - \alpha)(\beta - \alpha)}\right] = \frac{116}{3.01} = 38.54 \tag{14.72}$$

$$Q = \frac{B}{k_a} = \frac{FD}{V_1}\left[\frac{(k_{21} - \beta)}{(k_a - \beta)(\alpha - \beta)}\right] = \frac{27.1}{3.01} = 9.00 \tag{14.73}$$

$$R = \frac{C'}{k_a} = \frac{FD}{V_1}\left[\frac{(k_{21} - k_a)}{(\alpha - k_a)(\beta - k_a)}\right] = -\frac{143}{3.01} = -47.51 \tag{14.74}$$

From Equations 14.72 and 14.73, the relationships in Equations 14.75 and 14.76, respectively, can be derived.

$$FD/V_1 = P(k_a - \alpha) + Q(k_a - \beta) \tag{14.75}$$

$$V_1 = FD/[P(k_a - \alpha) + Q(k_a - \beta)] \tag{14.76}$$

Equation 14.76 provides an expression for the volume of the central compartment in this model. However, as in the oral absorption case for the one-compartment model, solving for V_1 is not always possible unless the value for F, the fraction of administered drug absorbed into the systemic circulation, is known.

To solve for the three microscopic rate constants, a little additional information is needed. The area under the plasma profile can be obtained by integrating Equation 14.66 between the limits of zero and infinite time to obtain

$$AUC^{0 \to \infty} = A/\alpha + B/\beta + C'/k_a \tag{14.77}$$

The same area can be obtained, however, by integrating Equation 14.65 between the same limits, and canceling like terms to obtain

$$\text{AUC}^{0 \to \infty} = D/(V_1 k_{el}) \tag{14.78}$$

Equations 14.77 and 14.78 can be combined to form Equation 14.79.

$$V_1 k_{el} = \frac{D}{\dfrac{A}{\alpha} + \dfrac{B}{\beta} + \dfrac{C'}{k_a}} \tag{14.79}$$

Substitution from Equations 14.72, 14.73, and 14.74 for A, B, and C' in Equation 14.79 yields

$$V_1 k_{el} = D/[(Pk_a/\alpha) + (Qk_a/\beta) + R] \tag{14.80}$$

Taking reciprocals of both sides of this equation, using Equation 14.79 to solve for V_1, and using the relationship in Equation 14.81 yields Equation 14.82.

$$k_{el} = \alpha\beta/k_{21} \tag{14.81}$$

$$k_{21} = \frac{\beta k_a P + \alpha k_a Q + \alpha\beta R}{P(k_a - \alpha) + Q(k_a - \beta)} \tag{14.82}$$

which yields the first of the three microscopic rate constants. Because k_{21} is solved, the other two constants are readily obtained from Equations 14.81 and 14.83.

$$k_{12} = \alpha + \beta - k_{21} - k_{el} \tag{14.83}$$

The numerical values for these calculations are given in Equations 14.84, 14.85, and 14.86.

$$k_{21} = \frac{(0.06)(3.01)(38.54) + (1.33)(3.01)(9.0) - (1.33)(0.06)(47.51)}{38.54(3.01 - 1.33) + 9.0(3.01 - 0.06)}$$

$$\tag{14.84}$$

$$k_{el} = [(1.33)\ (0.06)]/0.43 = 0.185 \qquad (14.85)$$

$$k_{12} = 1.33 + 0.06 - 0.43 - 0.185 = 0.775 \qquad (14.86)$$

Some Model-Independent Parameters for a Drug that Obeys Two-Compartment Model Kinetics

In Chapter 1, three approaches to pharmacokinetics were described: the compartment model approach, the physiological model approach, and the model-independent approach. The one-compartment model, being the simplest way in which drug disposition can be described, is really a model-independent method.

The use of true model-independent kinetics becomes particularly useful when dealing with compounds that obey multicompartment kinetics, for example, the two-compartment model. The two-compartment model with intravenous injection will be used to illustrate the model-independent approach.

The blood-level curve in Figure 14.1 was previously described in shorthand notation by Equation 14.12. If further interpretation of this equation (i.e., as in Equation 14.11) is avoided, then model-independent kinetics is being applied. The drug-level curve is being described by a biexponential equation that has two coefficients (or concentration terms) A and B, and two rate constants (α and β). The volume term in Equation 14.20, the terminal half-life in Equation 14.28, the area under the drug-concentration curve in Equation 14.31, and the plasma clearance in Equation 14.33 were obtained from the four parameters A, B, α, and β. In other words, these equations were based on a simple biexponential equation and are therefore completely model-independent.

Thus, a great deal of information can be obtained about a drug by the model-independent approach. Whether the model-dependent or model-independent approach is used depends entirely on the type of study, the questions being asked, and the quality of the data.

Although calculating pharmacokinetic parameters using a model-independent approach is quite simple, one parameter, the overall drug distribution volume at steady state, is more difficult to obtain. This parameter is useful because it describes, in a model-independent manner, the distribution characteristics of a drug that has equilibrated into the various tissues and body fluids.

The first solution to this problem was described by Wagner (11), who showed that the value V_{dss} can be obtained from

$$V_{dss} = \text{dose}\ \frac{\Sigma(A_i/\lambda_i^2)}{[\Sigma(A_i/\lambda_i)]^2} \qquad (14.87)$$

where A is a concentration term and λ is a rate constant. For the biexponential intravenous case (Equation 14.12) Equation 14.87 can be written as Equation 14.88.

$$V_{dss} = \text{dose } [(A/\alpha^2) + (B/\beta^2)]/[(A/\alpha) + (B/\beta)]^2 \qquad (14.88)$$

An alternative solution was described by Benet and Galeazzi (12). This approach provides a method to calculate V_{dss} that is model and rate constant-independent. The derivation of the method is not included here, but the final expression is

$$V_{dss} = \text{dose}[AUMC^{0\to\infty}]/[AUC^{0\to\infty}]^2 \qquad (14.89)$$

This equation yields V_{dss} as a function of the administered dose, the area under the moment curve (AUMC), and the square of the area under the blood-level curve. The area under the moment curve is given by

$$AUMC^{0\to\infty} = \int_0^\infty tC \cdot dt \qquad (14.90)$$

which is simply the area under the curve of the product of time and plasma concentration from zero to infinite time. The AUMC can be considered to be the sum of the residence times of all drug molecules in the body from the time of administration to the time when all drug molecules have left the body.

Summary

1. For many drugs, particularly after bolus intravenous administration, a multicompartment model provides a more accurate description of drug plasma profiles than a one-compartment kinetic model. The multicompartment is frequently represented by a two-compartment kinetic model.

2. With the two-compartment kinetic model, drug concentration profiles in plasma are characterized by an α phase of fast decline and a β phase of slower decline.

3. Initial graphical estimates can be used to obtain values of microscopic disposition constants associated with the two-compartment model.

4. A variety of methods have been described to obtain the overall equilibrium distribution volume for a drug that obeys two-compartment model kinetics. Only one of these V_{dss} is a true constant. Other constants are influenced by the relative magnitudes of mi-

croscopic elimination and disposition constants, and may yield biased values.

5. For a drug that obeys two-compartment model kinetics, the ratio of drug in the tissue compartment to that in plasma is a function of the distribution rate constants and the drug elimination rate.

6. Estimates of pharmacokinetic parameters can be obtained from urinary excretion data by use of sigma-minus plots.

7. Plasma drug profiles after oral administration of a drug that obeys two-compartment model kinetics are triexponential. The curves are characterized by absorption, α, and β phases.

8. Estimates of kinetic parameters can be obtained by standard curve-stripping procedures. Values of microscopic rate constants may be derived from initial estimates of components of the triexponential function.

9. Values of many pharmacokinetic parameters, including the equilibrium distribution volume, can be obtained by model-independent methods.

Literature Cited

1. Riegelman, S; Loo, J. C. K; Rowland, M. *J. Pharm. Sci.,* **1968,** *57,* 117–123.
2. Mayersohn, M.; Gibaldi, M. *Am. J. Pharm. Ed.,* **1971,** *35,* 19–28.
3. Rescigno, A.; Segre, G. *Drug and Tracer Kinetics;* Blaisdell Publishing: Waltham, MA, 1966, pp 24, 91.
4. O'Reilly, R. A.; Welling, P. G.; Wagner, J. G. *Thrombos. Diath. Hemorrhag.,* **1971,** *25,* 178–186.
5. Wagner, J. G. *J. Pharmacokinet. Biopharm.,* **1975,** *3,* 457–478.
6. Riegelman, S.; Loo, J. C. K; Rowland, M. *J. Pharm. Sci.,* **1968,** *57,* 128–133.
7. Jusko, W. J.; Gibaldi, M. *J. Pharm. Sci.,* **1972,** *61,* 1270–1273.
8. Benet, L. Z. *J. Pharm Sci.,* **1972,** *61,* 536–541.
9. Kaplan, S. A.; Jack, M. L; Alexander, K.; Weinfeld, R. E. *J. Pharm. Sci.,* **1973,** *62,* 1789–1796.
10. Welling, P. G.; Lee, K. P.; Patel, J. A.; Walker, J. A.; Wagner, J. G. *J. Pharm Sci.,* **1971,** *60,* 1629–1634.
11. Wagner, J. G. *J. Pharmacokinet. Biopharm.,* **1976,** *4,* 443–467.
12. Benet, L. Z.; Galeazzi, R. L. *J. Pharm. Sci.,* **1979,** *68,* 1071–1074.

Problems

1. A drug (200 mg) was administered to a patient by bolus intravenous injection. The decline in log plasma concentrations of unchanged drug was biphasic, and the half-life of the terminal linear elimination phase was 6.9 h. By curve stripping, the following values of microscopic rate constants were found: $k_{12} = 0.6$ h^{-1}, $k_{21} = 0.4$ h^{-1}, and $k_{el} = 0.3$ h^{-1}. The concentration of unchanged drug in plasma immediately after injection (allowing 1–2 min for

mixing) was 40 μg/mL. Total excretion of unchanged drug in urine accounted for 55% of the dose; the rest of the dose was metabolized. Calculate the following: (i) $V_{d\beta}$, (ii) $V_{d(extrap)}$, (iii) V_{dss}, (iv) plasma clearance, and (v) renal clearance.

2. Given that a drug obeys two-compartment model kinetics, and that the disposition rate constants, k_{12} and k_{21}, have values of 0.37 h^{-1} and 0.25 h^{-1}, respectively, calculate the shortest possible biological half-life of the drug.

3. Following a rapid intravenous dose of 500 mg of cefotaxime to a patient with normal renal function, plasma levels of unchanged drug declined in a biphasic manner, and the following parameter values were obtained: $A = 50$ μg/mL, $B = 15$ μg/mL, $\alpha = 3.5\ h^{-1}$, $\beta = 0.6\ h^{-1}$. What is the plasma clearance of cefotaxime?

4. From the data in problem 3, calculate the terminal-phase elimination half-life of cefotaxime.

5. Are plasma concentrations of a drug that obeys two-compartment model kinetics following an oral dose (i) monophasic, (ii) biphasic, or (iii) triphasic?

6. Mathematical analysis of the plasma levels in problem 5 yielded the following expression: $C = 59e^{-1.2t} + 130e^{-0.32t} - 189e^{-3.1t}$. What is the drug terminal elimination half-life?

7. From the data in problem 6, what is the area under the plasma curve from zero to infinite time?

8. If the drug dose leading to the plasma levels described in problem 6 was 100 mg, and the drug was 80% available to the systemic circulation, what is the plasma clearance?

9. Suppose the drug described in problem 6 was cleared 75% as unchanged drug via the kidneys, and the balance by hepatic metabolism. What are (i) the renal clearance, and (ii) the hepatic clearance?

15

Physiological Pharmacokinetic Models

The major focus in the preceding chapters has been on the classical compartment-based pharmacokinetic model. The simplifying assumptions in that model were that drugs or metabolites distribute into one or more body compartments, and that movement of drug between compartments, and also elimination from the body, can be described by one or more first-order processes.

These types of kinetic models are simple approximations and tend to serve a descriptive function, usually with regard to drug profiles in plasma or urinary excretion. These types of models do not attempt to address the more specific and often intractable problems that relate to the actual time course of drug or metabolite disposition in particular body organs and tissues.

Physiological Pharmacokinetic Model Description

One approach that has attempted to address these problems is based on the physiological model, in which the body is divided into compartments based on true anatomical regions or volumes such as blood, heart, liver, and central nervous system. The time course of drug or metabolite levels in the various "physiological" organs or compartments is calculated on the basis of blood flow rate through each particular region, diffusion of drug between blood and tissue, and the relative affinity of drug for blood and the various tissues and organs.

0065-7719/86/0185-0241$06.00/1
© 1986 American Chemical Society

Because of the large number of parameters that are involved in these studies, physiological models are necessarily more complicated than the classical compartment models considered previously. Complications are such that physiological models have been developed for very few drugs and are justified only to investigate specific tissue localization of drugs such as anticancer agents, or to examine the detailed mechanisms of drug metabolism or excretion by the liver, kidney, lung, or other organ.

Thus, physiological models have some advantages and some disadvantages compared with the compartment model approach. The principal advantages are:

1. Pharmacokinetic parameters are realistic because they are based on observed or predicted physiological values.

2. Parameter values can be altered to allow for changes in physiological function.

3. Total, free, and bound compound concentration profiles can be predicted for selected regions of the body.

4. Insight can be obtained regarding specific organ elimination mechanisms.

5. Parameter values can be "scaled" for different animal species and humans.

The advantages of the physiological model approach may be summarized briefly in that this model provides more information based on specific tissue localization and handling of compounds, and is particularly useful for some drugs.

The principal disadvantages of the physiological model approach are as follows:

1. The models are complicated; their mathematics are often difficult to solve.

2. It is difficult to validate a physiological model in animals and virtually impossible in humans because large numbers of tissue samples are required at different time intervals after dosing.

3. It is difficult to obtain tissue samples that are free of blood.

4. Model development requires a large data base for each drug or drug group in a particular species.

5. In vitro testing is frequently required to establish or validate model parameters.

6. Despite their complexity, physiological models often contain many simplifying assumptions regarding diffusion of drug into tissues,

complete mixing within organs, and the relative degree of intravascular and extravascular drug binding.

The disadvantages may thus be summarized in the following manner. Considerable information is needed to develop the model; the model still contains many assumptions, certainly of a more microscopic nature than the comparatively gross assumptions associated with the compartmental approach; the model is often difficult, sometimes impossible, to validate; and species differences may also cause complications.

On a more general note, the development and validation of physiological models, whether successful or not, can only help to improve the understanding of the rates and mechanisms of drug absorption, distribution, metabolism, and excretion, whether the work is carried out in vivo or in situ with animal models, or in vitro in isolated organ systems. At the very worst this approach increases understanding of the processes involved. At best the approach may facilitate more rigorous characterization of drug pharmacokinetic and pharmacodynamic properties than can be obtained by other model systems.

Before discussing some aspects of physiological pharmacokinetic models, it is important to understand the concept of organ clearance, which is a fundamental component for this type of model.

Organ Clearance

Possibly the best way to understand organ clearance is to consider a single organ that is well perfused by the bloodstream and is capable of eliminating the drug. This simple model, with or without the elimination component, provides the basic building block of physiological pharmacokinetic models. The model is shown in Scheme 15.1. The symbol Q represents blood flow rate through the organ, and C_i and C_o represent

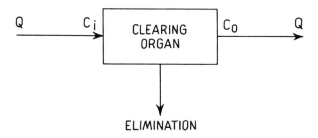

Scheme 15.1. Physiological flow model for a well-perfused organ that is capable of drug elimination.

drug concentrations in blood entering and leaving the organ, respectively. If an eliminating organ is considered, then $C_i > C_o$.

The rate that blood introduces drug to the organ is equal to the blood flow rate multiplied by the drug concentration:

$$\text{rate of drug entry into organ in blood} = QC_i \qquad (15.1)$$

Because Q has units of volume per unit time and C_i has units of mass per volume, the product of Q and C_i has units of mass per unit time. If drug is eliminated by the organ, then the rate that drug leaves the organ is similarly equal to the blood flow rate, Q, multiplied by the drug concentration, C_o:

$$\text{rate at which drug leaves organ in blood} = QC_o \qquad (15.2)$$

The difference between the rate of drug entry into the organ and the rate that drug leaves the organ is accounted for by the rate of eliminated drug:

$$\text{drug elimination rate} = QC_i - QC_o = Q(C_i - C_o) \qquad (15.3)$$

This type of expression, flow rate multiplied by the concentration difference, is commonly used to denote organ clearance, which has units of mass per unit time. This expression is useful because it indicates how much of the drug the organ can eliminate in a certain time period. However, in Chapter 9, clearance was described in terms of the volume of plasma cleared of drug per unit time. Clearance due to particular organs was also defined in terms of the volume of plasma cleared of drug by that particular organ, for example, renal clearance and hepatic clearance. Describing organ clearance with the same units in the physiological model is possible. To do this, the organ extraction ratio, E, needs to be defined. This ratio compares the rate of drug elimination with the rate that drug enters the organ:

$$E = [Q(C_i - C_o)]/QC_i = (C_i - C_o)/C_i \qquad (15.4)$$

The organ extraction ratio is a dimensionless quantity. This ratio indicates how efficiently the organ removes drug from the bloodstream. If removal is very inefficient and removes essentially no drug, then C_o will equal C_i, and the extraction ratio is zero. On the other hand, if removal is very efficient and removes all of the drug as it passes through the organ, then C_o is zero, and the extraction ratio is unity. For most eliminating organs, the extraction ratio lies somewhere between these two extremes. For example, an extraction ratio of 0.45 indicates that 45% of the blood flowing through the organ is completely cleared of the drug. Thus, the organ clearance in this case will be 45% of the blood flow rate through the organ. This relationship is described by

$$Cl_{or} = [Q(C_i - C_o)]/C_i = QE \tag{15.5}$$

In this case, the organ clearance, Cl_{or}, has units of volume of blood cleared of drug per unit time. Thus, to express organ clearance in the same units as plasma clearance established in Chapter 9, the blood flow rate must be multiplied by the extraction ratio. If all of the individual organ clearances are added together, the total body clearance, or plasma clearance, is obtained. The terms body clearance and plasma clearance are generally used synonymously.

Blood Flow Rate-Limited Transport

A physiological pharmacokinetic model consists of a series of body tissues or organs linked by blood flow in a pattern that approximates or simulates the true anatomical and physiological situation. An example of this type of model is shown in Scheme 15.2. The choice of organs to be included in a model depends on anatomical and physiological reality and on the characteristics and site of action of the drug to be examined. Typically, organs where the compound exerts its pharmacological activity (i.e., organs that contain or accumulate large quantities of drug) and organs involved in drug elimination would be included.

   When a drug in the bloodstream reaches an organ, the drug cannot enter the cells of that organ directly, but must pass through the capillary membranes into interstitial fluid, and then through the membrane separating interstitial fluid from the organ or tissue cells. This process is illustrated in Scheme 15.3. It is often assumed that drug transport across these membranes is very fast, that drug distribution into a specific organ is limited only by blood flow rate into that organ, and also that the concentration of drug in the emergent or venous blood from a particular organ is in equilibrium with the drug concentration in the intracellular fluid in that organ. This description is the essence of the blood flow rate- or perfusion-limited model, which permits organs to be represented by a simple, single compartment as illustrated in Scheme 15.3. This approach is suitable for any molecule that readily and rapidly crosses membranes. These molecules include only partially ionized or un-ionized fat-soluble compounds.

   For ionized or water-soluble compounds, the assumption of very rapid equilibrium across physiological membranes may be inappropriate. Membrane transport will probably be slow, and rapid equilibrium cannot

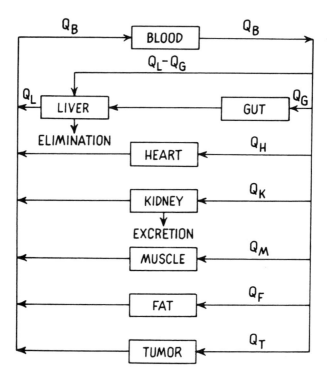

Scheme 15.2. A general physiological pharmacokinetic model. Q denotes blood flow rate to a region. Subscripts are as follows: B, blood; L, liver; G, gut; H, heart; K, kidney; M, muscle; F, fat; and T, tumor. Elimination occurs from the liver and kidney.

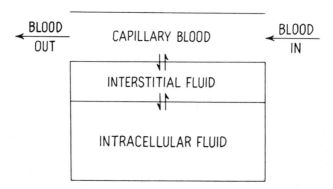

Scheme 15.3. Model of drug transport between blood and intracellular fluid; this is the blood flow rate-limiting model.

be assumed. This situation is recognized in the membrane-limited model that will be discussed later.

Most whole body physiological models are complex and are similar to the model shown in Scheme 15.2. However, to understand how the appropriate mathematical expressions are derived, consider two small subunits, one consisting of blood and a noneliminating organ such as muscle, the other consisting of blood and an eliminating organ such as the kidney. These subunits are illustrated in Scheme 15.4. In Model A

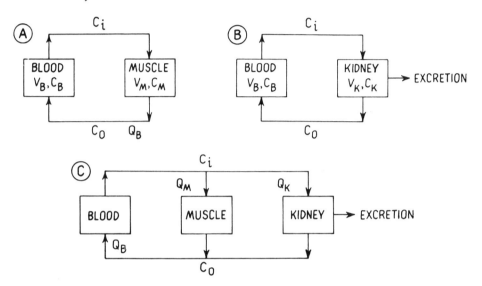

Scheme 15.4. Physiological flow models representing (A) blood and muscle, (B) blood and kidney, and (C) blood, muscle, and kidney. Q_X is blood flow rate through organ X, V is volume of organ. Subscripts are as follows: B, blood; M, muscle; and K, kidney. C_i is drug concentration in arterial (afferent) blood, and C_o is drug concentration in venous (efferent) blood.

of this scheme, the rates of change in the total drug concentration in the blood pool, C_B, and also in the muscle, C_M, may be represented by the difference in drug concentration in the blood that flows through each tissue or fluid volume. The rates of change of total drug in blood and muscle are represented by Equations 15.6 and 15.7, respectively.

$$V_B \, (dC_B/dt) = Q_M C_o - Q_M C_i = Q_M(C_o - C_i) \qquad (15.6)$$

$$V_M \, (dC_M/dt) = Q_M C_i - Q_M C_o = Q_M(C_i - C_o) \qquad (15.7)$$

In these equations, V_B and V_M are the volumes of the blood and muscle compartments, respectively; Q_M represents blood flow through muscle; and C_i and C_o are the entering, or afferent, and exiting, or efferent, blood drug concentrations. In these models, the drug concentration in entering blood, C_i, is equivalent to arterial drug concentration, C_B, and the drug concentration in exiting blood, C_o, is equal to C_M if no binding in blood or muscle occurs, or if binding in blood and muscle is identical, which is unlikely. If unequal binding occurs, or some other situation exists that prevents C_o being exactly equal to C_M, then

$$C_o = C_M / R_M \tag{15.8}$$

where R_M is the partition coefficient for distribution of drug from blood into tissue at equilibrium. Again the assumption is made that blood leaving the tissue is in equilibrium with drug within the tissue. Clearly, if $R_M = 2$, then the total drug concentration in tissue is double that in blood, and $C_o = 1/2\ C_M$. Equation 15.8 can also be expressed as

$$R_M = C_M / C_o \tag{15.9}$$

The concentration of total drug in a tissue compartment is equal to the free concentration multiplied by the free fraction. That is, if the free fraction is 10 µg/mL and the drug is 50% free, then the total concentration is 20 µg/mL. In that case, R_M can be described in terms of the relative free fractions of drug in blood, f_B, and tissue, f_M, by

$$R_M = f_B / f_M \tag{15.10}$$

Assume that a drug is extensively bound to muscle protein, and the free fraction in muscle is only 20%, while the drug is bound to only a small extent in blood, and the fraction free in blood is 80%. In this case, R_M is equal to 0.8/0.2, which equals 4. In other words, the concentration of total drug in the muscle compartment is four times greater than efferent, or exiting blood, at equilibrium. Taking this into account, Equations 15.6 and 15.7 can be rewritten as Equations 15.11 and 15.12.

$$V_B(dC_B/dt) = Q_M(C_M/R_M) - Q_M C_B = Q_M[(C_M/R_M) - C_B] \tag{15.11}$$

$$V_M(dC_M/dt) = Q_M C_B - Q_M(C_M/R_M) = Q_M[C_B - (C_M/R_M)] \tag{15.12}$$

In these equations, the drug concentrations in afferent and efferent blood are more specifically identified in relation to the drug concentrations in tissue and the partitioning of drug from blood into tissue.

When drug distribution into an eliminating organ is considered, the elimination process has to be taken into account. Therefore, in Model B of Scheme 15.4, the equivalent equations to 15.6 and 15.7 for blood and kidney tissue, respectively, are Equations 15.13 and 15.14.

$$V_B(dC_B/dt) = Q_KC_o - Q_KC_i = Q_K(C_o - C_i) \tag{15.13}$$

$$V_K(dC_K/dt) = Q_KC_i - Q_KC_o - Cl_KC_K \tag{15.14}$$

where V_K is the volume of the kidney, Q_K is the blood flow through the kidney, and Cl_K is the clearance of drug by the kidney. If the drug is partially bound in the kidney, and only free drug is cleared, then the term Cl_KC_K, which represents the rate of drug removal by the kidney, would be replaced by $Cl'_KC'_K$, where the primes denote the free drug clearance and the free drug concentration, respectively. Equations 15.13 and 15.14 can also be converted to Equations 15.15 and 15.16 in terms of total drug concentrations in the blood and kidney compartments.

$$V_B(dC_B/dt) = Q_K[(C_K/R_K) - C_B] \tag{15.15}$$

$$V_K(dC_K/dt) = Q_K[C_B - (C_K/R_K)] - Cl_KC_K \tag{15.16}$$

Thus, expressions have been derived that describe the rates of change in drug concentrations in blood and tissue for the situations in Models A and B of Figure 15.1. These expressions can now be combined to obtain overall expressions for the more complete situation in Model C of Scheme 15.4, that is, for the combined Models A and B. Drug in blood, muscle, and kidney is represented by the rate Equations 15.17, 15.18, and 15.19, respectively.

$$V_B(dC_B/dt) = Q_M(C_M/R_M) + Q_K(C_K/R_K) - Q_BC_B \tag{15.17}$$

$$V_M(dC_M/dt) = Q_M[C_B - (C_M/R_M)] \tag{15.18}$$

$$V_K(dC_K/dt) = Q_K[C_B - (C_K/R_K)] - Cl_KC_K \tag{15.19}$$

Equation 15.17, the rate equation for drug in blood, is now expanded to include the input terms from both muscle and kidney.

Equations 15.17–15.19 are thus a complete set of rate equations for Model C of Scheme 15.4. From this relatively simple example, construction of a similar set of equations for more complex models, such as the one in Scheme 15.2, is not difficult (1). The liver compartment in that model, with its dual blood input from the systemic and splanchnic circulations, is representative of the true anatomical situation, and the rate of change of total drug concentration in liver in that model is given by

$$V_L(dC_L/dt) = C_B(Q_L - Q_G) + Q_G(C_G/R_G) - Q_L(C_L/R_L) - Cl_LC_L \tag{15.20}$$

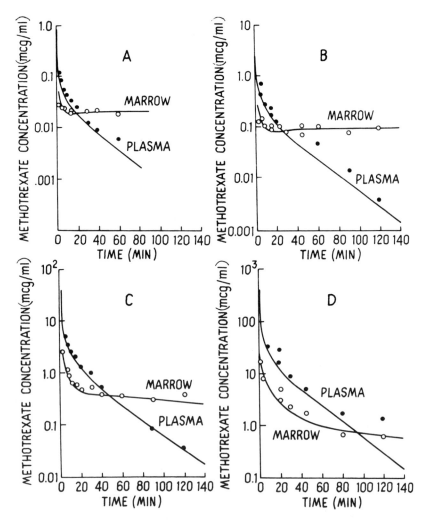

Figure 15.1. Plasma and average bone-marrow concentrations of methotrexate in the rat. Solid lines represent model simulations. Data points were obtained from one rat each time. Key (mg/kg IV): A, 0.05; B, 0.25 C, 2.5; and D, 25. (Reproduced with permission from Ref. 4. Copyright 1973, American Pharmaceutical Association.)

In these examples, drug distribution into body tissues and fluids is assumed to be limited by blood flow rate. This limit is generally the case, but not always. Some compounds, for example, water-soluble compounds, methotrexate, and actinomycin D, have tissue uptake characteristics that are not consistent with the simple blood flow model (2–4). Typically, the relationships between concentrations of these compounds in blood and in certain tissues are not simple or linear. These drugs behave as though there were some barrier preventing rapid equilibrium. One way of interpreting these types of situations incorporates the concept of membrane-limited transport.

Membrane-Limited Transport

A typical tissue model for membrane-limited transport between blood and organ tissue is shown in Scheme 15.5. This model is different from the one in Scheme 15.3 because the membrane barrier between interstitial fluid and intracellular fluid has increased and is now rate-limiting.

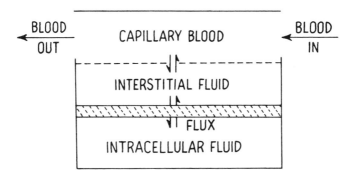

Scheme 15.5. Model of drug transport between blood and intracellular fluid; this is the membrane-limited transport model.

The net flux, or drug transport, across this limiting membrane may be controlled by passive diffusion or by a Michaelis–Menten-type process (4,5). (Michaelis–Menten processes will be described in greater detail in Chapter 16.)

Whenever drug metabolism or drug movement from one place to the other, for example, across membranes into cells, is dependent upon an enzymatic or active transport process, then a likelihood of Michaelis–Menten, or saturable kinetics, exists. In Michaelis–Menten kinetics, the constants that characterize a saturable reaction are V_m (or V_{max}), which is the maximum rate of a reaction, and K_m, the Michaelis constant, which is the substrate concentration at which the rate is one-half the maximum value V_m. Thus, at high drug concentrations (the actual concentration depending on the efficiency of the particular process) the enzyme or transporting agent can become saturated. Although leading to first-order kinetics at low drug concentrations, this process may become less efficient at high drug concentrations, and the rate of the particular event becomes limited by the availability of enzyme or carrier; apparent zero-order kinetics results.

For diffusion transport, which has been shown to occur, for example with actinomycin D uptake by dog testes, net flux across the limiting membrane is given by

$$\text{flux} = K(C_E - C_I) \tag{15.21}$$

where K is the membrane permeability coefficient, and C_E and C_I represent extracellular and intracellular drug concentrations, respectively. If drug movement across the membrane is saturable, then Equation 15.21 needs to be expanded to include the Michaelis–Menten functions:

$$\text{flux} = K(C_E - C_I) + [V_M C_E/(K_M + C_E)] - [V_M C_I/(K_M + C_I)] \tag{15.22}$$

Michaelis–Menten functions have been included in both directions because active transport may occur both for drug movement into and out of the cell.

Incorporating these membrane-limited transport expressions into overall physiological models is difficult. More parameters have been introduced for which initial estimates have to be obtained, and the complexity and therefore the uncertainty of the model are increased. This type of approach nonetheless has been used successfully to describe methotrexate kinetics. Figure 15.1 illustrates the close agreement that has been obtained between predicted and observed methotrexate levels in bone marrow and plasma of rats using the membrane-limited model (4).

Experimental Considerations

Discussion so far has been limited to some of the theory relating to physiological pharmacokinetic models. But how are the models used in practice? The most common approach is to set up the model that is thought to be most appropriate for the system to be studied; substitute in estimates for the constants involved, for example, blood flow rates, organ volumes, and binding parameters; and solve the equations simultaneously as a function of time to establish theoretical concentration versus time plots in the sites of interest. Introduction of drug into the model is usually done as a program step. For example, an intravenous bolus injection is an initial condition in the blood pool, whereas an intramuscular injection is introduced as an initial condition in muscle. Similarly, intrathecal injection is an initial condition in cerebrospinal fluid.

Once the model is validated (if this can be done), it can be used to predict drug disposition in humans under a variety of dosing conditions, provided that animal data can be successfully applied to humans for that particular drug and situation (6,7).

The blood flow rates and tissue volumes used are generally average values for a particular species. Most of these, under normal conditions, are available in the literature. However, drugs are often given under disease conditions, and drug may also affect the physiological conditions because of pharmacological actions. These factors can perturb the model and lead to difficulty in interpretation. Some typical tissue volumes and blood flow rates in humans are given in Table 15.1.

Table 15.1—Volumes and Blood Flow Rates

Region	Volume (L)	Blood Flow (mL/min)
Blood	5	—
Plasma	3	—
Muscle	30	1200
Kidneys	0.3	1250
Liver	1.5	1500
Heart	0.3	240
GI tract	2.4	1200
Fat	10.0	200
Brain	1.5	750

NOTE: Values apply for a 70-kg male with body surface area of 1.82 m² and cardiac output of 5600 mL/min.

The very brief introduction to physiological kinetic modeling in this chapter has shown that this approach to pharmacokinetics is complex, and quite demanding experimentally. As indicated at the beginning of this chapter, this aproach is not of general application in most situations. The physiological model may be used to solve particular distribution problems for drugs when tissue distribution is important, or when sites of elimination are critical. Thus, the physiological model applies naturally to anticancer compounds and drugs acting on the central nervous system. Most of the published work has been done in these areas.

Summary

1. Physiological pharmacokinetic models, unlike classical compartment models, are based on true anatomical regions and volumes, blood flow rate through these regions, and transport of drug between blood and tissue.

2. Physiological pharmacokinetic models have advantages and disadvantages compared with compartment models. Advantages are associated with more accurate characterization of drug disposition. Disadvantages are associated with model complexity and difficulty in validation.

3. Physiological models are particularly useful for compounds such as anticancer agents when drug location in specific organs is important.

4. Drug transport from blood to organ tissue may be limited by blood flow rate or by the rate that drug diffuses between blood and tissue.

5. Diffusion- or membrane-limited transport may be controlled by passive diffusion or by saturable, active transport processes.

6. The predictability of physiological models is influenced by species differences and disease states that can affect physiological conditions.

Literature Cited

1. Himmelstein, K. J.; Lutz, R. J. *J. Pharmacokinet. Biopharm.*, **1979**, *7*, 127–145.
2. Lutz, R. J.; Galbraith, W. M.; Dedrick, R. L.; Shrager, R.; Mellett, L. B. *J. Pharmacol. Exp. Ther.*, **1971**, *200*, 469–478.
3. Bischoff, K. B.; Dedrick, R. L.; Zaharko, D. S.; Longstreth, J. A. *J. Pharm. Sci.*, **1971**, *60*, 1128–1133.
4. Dedrick, R. L.; Zaharko, D. S.; Lutz, R. J. *J. Pharm. Sci.*, **1973**, *62*, 882–890.
5. Mintun, M.; Himmelstein, K. J.; Schroder, R. L.; Gibaldi, M.; Shen, D. D. *J. Pharmacokinet. Biopharm.*, **1980**, *8*, 373–409.
6. Dedrick, R. L. *J. Pharmacokinet. Biopharm.*, **1973**, *1*, 435–461.
7. Dedrick, R. L.; Bischoff, K. B. *Fed. Proc.*, **1980**, *39*, 54–59.

Problems

1. The blood concentration of drug entering the kidneys via the renal arteries is 8 μg/mL. The blood concentration of drug leaving the kidneys via the renal veins is 5 μg/mL. If blood flow to the kidneys is 1200 mL/min, what are (i) the kidney extraction ratio and (ii) the renal clearance?

2. If the drug concentration in blood entering the kidneys is 8 μg/mL and the drug concentration in blood leaving the kidney is zero, what is the kidney extraction ratio for the drug?

3. Blood flows through a particular noneliminating muscle tissue at a rate of 450 mL/min. Drug concentration is 9 μg/mL in afferent blood and 4 μg/mL in efferent blood. The partition coefficient for drug distribution from blood to muscle tissue is 1.5. Calculate the concentration of drug in muscle tissue.

4. What would the concentration of drug in muscle tissue be if the drug in problem 3 was 70% bound to blood proteins?

5. A drug that does not bind to plasma proteins or enter red cells is cleared by hepatic metabolism. A patient with a hematocrit of 0.44 has a hepatic blood flow of 1.5 L/min. If the hepatic extraction ratio for the drug is 0.4, and the drug level in afferent blood is 12.5 μg/mL, what are (i) the hepatic drug clearance, (ii) the concentration of drug in efferent blood, and (iii) the concentration of drug in efferent plasma?

16

Nonlinear Pharmacokinetics

Despite the wide diversity of the classical and physiological pharmacokinetic models, all of these models, with the exception of the membrane-limited transport model discussed in Chapter 15, incorporate the common assumption that drug elimination from the body is a first-order process. Another incorporated assumption is that the rate constant for elimination is a true constant and is independent of drug concentration. In these cases, the rate that drug is cleared from the body is concentration dependent, the percentage of body drug load that is cleared per unit time is constant, and the drug has an elimination half-life.

Saturable Processes

Fortunately, first-order elimination, or apparent first-order elimination, is common. First-order elimination greatly simplifies dosage design and adjustment, prediction of drug accumulation, bioavailability assessment, dose-response relationships, and a variety of other aspects of pharmacokinetics.

In fact, very few drugs are eliminated from the body by mechanisms that are truly first-order in nature. True first-order elimination applies only to compounds that are eliminated exclusively by mechanisms that do not involve enzymatic or transport processes, that is, any processes that involve energy. This elimination applies only to drugs that are cleared from the body by urinary excretion, and among those, only drugs that enter the renal tubule by glomerular filtration. All other processes require some form of energy-consuming metabolism or transport and are there-

0065-7719/86/0185-0255$06.00/1
© 1986 American Chemical Society

fore saturable. These processes apply to drugs that are metabolized in the liver or any other organ in the body, cleared in the urine by active secretion, or cleared in the bile by a similar active process. Even compounds like riboflavin, bethanidine, cephaloridine, and cephapirin that may undergo capacity-limited reabsorption from the distal renal tubule back into the circulation are included in this group (1). Saturable elimination is therefore a potential condition for the great majority of compounds. Of course, drugs may be excreted in saliva, sweat, or even to a small extent in bile by passive processes; but these elimination routes generally account for such a small proportion of total eliminated drug that they are generally negligible.

Awareness of saturable processes influencing pharmacokinetics is steadily increasing, particularly in the area of saturable first-pass metabolism affecting drug absorption efficiency. The evolution of this field of research is such that nonlinear approaches to drug disposition may play a more significant role in the future.

Why is it that although the vast majority of drugs and other compounds are cleared from the body by saturable processes, most drugs exhibit first-order (or apparent first-order) elimination kinetics? The answer of course is that in most cases concentrations of drug in the bloodstream, or more correctly at the site of elimination, are well below those required to saturate the processes involved.

One notable exception to this explanation is ethyl alcohol. Alcohol is cleared from the body by oxidative metabolism at an apparent zero-order rate that is equivalent to about 12 oz of beer or 1 oz of liquor per hour (2,3). The opinion is often expressed that zero-order elimination is a unique property of ethyl alcohol that differentiates it from most other drugs that are cleared either entirely at a first-order rate, or at least at such a rate at low drug concentrations.

However, alcohol loses much of this uniqueness if one considers how much compound the body is being required to cope with. One bottle of eight-proof beer is equivalent to about 8 g of pure alcohol. The molecular weight of ethyl alcohol is 46, which is about one-quarter the molecular weight of aspirin, and much less than that of many drugs that are in the 200–400 molecular weight range. Thus, if an equivalent dose on a "per molecule" basis is considered, then the 8-g dose of ethyl alcohol is equivalent to 32 g of aspirin or 77 g of tetracycline. Ingestion of this quantity of any drug that is eliminated by a saturable pathway would yield apparent zero-order kinetics, or possibly no kinetics at all. In fact, administration of a sufficiently small dose of ethyl alcohol such that circulating levels are low relative to K_m for this compound yields first-order elimination kinetics (4).

Compounds such as phenytoin, salicylate, theophylline, probenecid, and possibly others that have not yet been examined carefully exhibit saturable kinetics within the therapeutic range (5–8). The most important of these drugs are phenytoin and salicylate. Phenytoin kinetics is usually interpreted as though its elimination proceeds via a single saturable pathway. Salicylate, on the other hand, forms a number of metabolites and formation of only two of these, salicyluric acid and salicylphenolic glucuronide, appears to be saturable. Thus, overall elimination of salicylate is best described in terms of parallel saturable and nonsaturable pathways (9,10).

As mentioned earlier, a constant percentage of a drug that is eliminated by first-order kinetics is cleared per unit time, and the drug has a discrete concentration-independent elimination half-life. For drugs that are eliminated by zero-order kinetics or by saturable pathways, however, the same quantity of drug is cleared per unit time, and this quantity is drug concentration-independent. Thus a different percentage of the drug is cleared per unit time depending on the concentration, and the drug does not have a constant, characteristic elimination half-life.

The difference between simple first-order elimination and saturable, leading ultimately to zero-order, elimination may have a profound effect on drug concentrations, the duration of drug activity, and the time course and extent of drug accumulation with repeated or continuous doses. Saturable hepatic metabolism may also markedly affect drug absorption because of altered first-pass metabolism.

Expressions Useful in Elimination Kinetics

As mentioned briefly in Chapter 15, saturable elimination of a compound, whether it be drug or metabolite, is generally described in the form of Michaelis–Menten kinetics.

For a drug that obeys one-compartment model kinetics, and whose elimination is first-order, the kinetic model following intravenous injection is given in Scheme 16.1, and the rate equation for loss of drug from the circulation with respect to time is given by Equation 16.1. The symbols for this model were described in Chapter 10.

$$dC/dt = -k_{el}C \qquad (16.1)$$

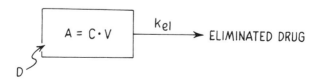

Scheme 16.1. One-compartment open model with first-order elimination after bolus intravenous injection.

where C is the concentration of drug in the body, k_{el} is the elimination rate constant, and t is time.

For a drug that is eliminated by a single saturable process, the kinetic model is given in Scheme 16.2, and the rate equation for loss of drug from the circulation is given by Equation 16.2.

$$dC/dt = -[V_m C/(K_m + C)] \tag{16.2}$$

where V_m is the maximum rate of elimination and K_m is the Michaelis constant.

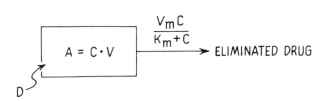

Scheme 16.2. One-compartment open model with a single route of saturable elimination after bolus intravenous injection.

The term on the right side of Equation 16.2 is a form of the familiar Michaelis–Menten expression for a saturable reaction based on a single substrate mechanism.

Typical drug profiles resulting from the models in Schemes 16.1 and 16.2 are shown on linear and semilogarithmic scales in Figure 16.1. The profiles in Figure 16.1A describe first-order loss of drug. The profiles in Figure 16.1B, however, describe Michaelis–Menten elimination. When the concentration in B is plotted on a linear scale, the decline in levels is initially linear or zero-order, but becomes curved or first-order at lower levels to yield the familiar hockey-stick shape. When the data are plotted on a semilogarithmic scale, the decline is initially curvilinear but becomes linear at lower concentrations.

Why does Figure 16.1B yield apparent zero-order kinetics at high drug levels and apparent first-order kinetics at low drug levels? Consider the two situations where the drug concentration C is much greater or much less than the Michaelis constant K_m. In the situation where C is much greater than K_m Equation 16.2 becomes

$$dC/dt = -(V_m C/C) = -V_m \tag{16.3}$$

In this equation, the rate of elimination becomes essentially zero-order.

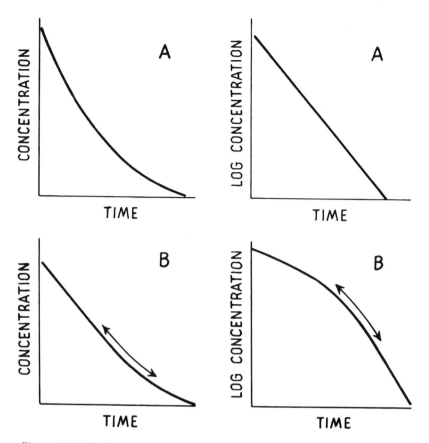

Figure 16.1. Blood concentration versus time profiles of a drug that is eliminated by first-order kinetics (A), and by Michaelis–Menten-type kinetics (B).

However, in the situation where C is much smaller than K_m, Equation 16.2 becomes

$$dC/dt = -(V_m C/K_m) = -kC \qquad (16.4)$$

The units of V_m/K_m are concentration per time per concentration, which cancels to reciprocal time. This unit is common for a first-order rate constant. Thus, in Equation 16.4, V_m/K_m can be expressed as a single apparent first-order rate constant, k.

In the region where the values of drug concentration and K_m are similar, Equation 16.2 is operative. This region is the transition state between the apparent first-order and apparent zero-order elimination regions. This region is identified by the arrows in Figure 16.1B.

Equation 16.2 can be expanded for various types of models. For example, the one-compartment model with first-order input and saturable elimination is represented by Equation 16.5, and the same model with zero-order drug input is given by Equation 16.6.

$$\frac{dC}{dt} = \frac{k_a FD}{V} e^{-k_{el}t} - \frac{V_m C}{K_m + C} \tag{16.5}$$

$$\frac{dC}{dt} = -k_0 V - \frac{V_m C}{K_m + C} \tag{16.6}$$

where F is the fraction of the dose, D, absorbed, and k_0 is the zero-order rate constant for drug input. If a drug is eliminated by both parallel saturable and nonsaturable pathways, then the rate equation after intravenous injection is given by

$$dC/dt = -k_{el}C - [V_m C/(K_m + C)] \tag{16.7}$$

If the drug obeys two-compartment model kinetics and is also cleared by both saturable and nonsaturable pathways, then referring back to Chapter 14, the rate equation for the amount of drug in the central compartment of that model after bolus intravenous injection is given by

$$dA_1/dt = k_{21}A_2 - (k_{12} + k_{el}) A_1 - [V_m A_1/(K_m + A_1)] \tag{16.8}$$

where A_1 and A_2 are the quantity of drug in the first compartment and the second compartment, respectively.

Writing the appropriate rate equations for the various situations is not difficult. However, obtaining initial estimates for the actual values of V_m and K_m, the Michaelis constants, is more difficult and requires good data. Several methods can be found in references 9–11. Two of these methods are described here.

Obtaining Estimates of V_m and K_m from Plasma-Level Data

The first method to obtain estimates of V_m and K_m from plasma data requires determination of the rate of change in plasma drug concentrations between successive sampling times during the postabsorptive and postdistributive phase of a plasma profile. Thus, the rate of change in plasma concentration, together with the drug concentration at the midpoint of each sampling period, C_m, can be incorporated into a number of expressions to solve for V_m and K_m.

A typical expression is

$$[1/(\Delta C/\Delta t)] = 1/V_m + (K_m/V_m)(1/C_m) \tag{16.9}$$

This equation is the Lineweaver–Burk expression, which is a linear form of the Michaelis–Menten equation. In this equation, $\Delta C/\Delta t$ and C_m represent the decline in drug concentrations during a time interval, and the drug concentration at the midpoint of the time interval, respectively. A plot of $1/(\Delta C/\Delta t)$ versus $1/C_m$ will thus yield a slope of K_m/V_m and an intercept of $1/V_m$, as in Figure 16.2.

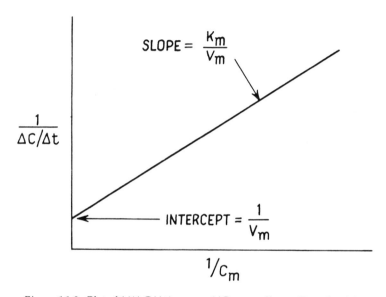

Figure 16.2. Plot of $1/(\Delta C/\Delta t)$ versus $1/C_m$ according to Equation 16.9.

In the second method, estimates of V_m and K_m are obtained directly from log C versus t data. Equation 16.2 can be rearranged to

$$-dC - [(K_m \cdot dC)/C] = V_m dt \tag{16.10}$$

Integration of Equation 16.10 yields

$$-C - K_m \ln C = V_m t + i \tag{16.11}$$

where i is the constant of integration. Solving for i at t equals zero, where C equals C_o, yields Equation 16.12.

$$i = -C_o - K_m \ln C_o \tag{16.12}$$

Substituting for i in Equation 16.11 gives

$$t = [(C_o - C)/V_m] + (K_m/V_m) \ln (C_o/C) \qquad (16.13)$$

Conversion of Equation 16.13 to logarithms to the base 10, and solving for log C yields

$$\log C = [(C_o - C)/2.3K_m] + \log C_o - (V_m t/2.3K_m) \qquad (16.14)$$

Consider log C versus t data following a bolus intravenous dose of a drug that obeys one-compartment model kinetics. The terminal log-linear portion of the log C versus t plot, that is, the region where apparent first-order kinetics occur, is a straight line described by

$$\log C = \log C_o^* - (V_m t/2.3K_m) \qquad (16.15)$$

where C_o^* is the extrapolated intercept of C on the y axis, as shown in Figure 16.3.

At low plasma concentrations in the log-linear region, Equation 16.15

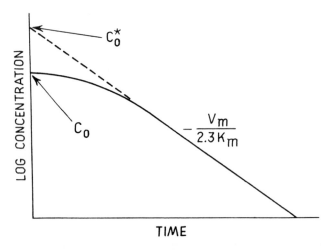

Figure 16.3. Estimates of V_m and K_m from a plot of log C versus t after bolus intravenous injection of a drug that obeys one-compartment model kinetics and undergoes saturable elimination.

is identical to Equation 16.14; therefore, the two expressions can be set equal:

$$\log C_o^* - \frac{V_m}{2.3K_m} t = \frac{C_o - C}{2.3K_m} + \log C_o - \frac{V_m t}{2.3K_m} \qquad (16.16)$$

Canceling the common term $V_m t/2.3K_m$ and rearranging yields

$$\log (C_o^*/C_o) = [(C_o - C)/2.3K_m] \qquad (16.17)$$

Because Equation 16.16 occurs only during the terminal linear phase of a drug profile, that is, when C is much less than C_o, the approximation that $(C_o - C) = C_o$ can be applied. Equation 16.17 then rearranges to

$$K_m = C_o/[2.3 \log (C_o^*/C_o)] = C_o/[\ln (C_o^*/C_o)] \qquad (16.18)$$

Because both C_o and C_o^*, the actual and extrapolated y intercepts, can be measured, K_m can be calculated from Equation 16.18, and V_m from Equation 16.19.

$$V_m = -2.3 \text{ (slope) } K_m \qquad (16.19)$$

The preceding are two of several possible ways to calculate Michaelis constants from plasma data. One method uses the rates of change in plasma concentrations, which may be based on either oral or intravenous data; the other method is based on direct estimates from plots of log plasma concentration versus time data, and is restricted to intravenous data.

A word of caution is appropriate regarding the fitting of saturable data to kinetic models, especially computer-fitting procedures. Equations of the type of 16.2, 16.5, and 16.6 are written as rate equations and have not been solved to yield expressions for drug concentration as a function of time because no analytical solution to these rate equations exists. Therefore, the rate equations must be used. During curve-fitting procedures, the computer carries out the necessary integration by means of numerical integration subroutines.

Influence of Saturable Kinetics on Drug Elimination, Area Under Drug Concentration Curve, and First-Pass Effect

Elimination Half-life. While blood concentrations of a drug are in the saturable range, the drug will not have a true half-life. The half-life will change continuously with drug concentration. The higher the drug concentration, the smaller the percentage cleared per unit time, and the longer the apparent half-life becomes. This phenomenon is particularly important with toxic drug overdoses when the levels of drug are most likely to be in the saturable range.

Although saturable elimination may thus profoundly affect the elimination of a drug that is cleared by one saturable process, a lesser effect may occur for the elimination of a drug that is cleared by parallel saturable and nonsaturable pathways. As drug concentrations are increased in this case, the apparent elimination half-life will tend to stabilize at a value larger than that observed at low drug concentrations. The apparent elimination half-life would nonetheless become concentration-independent because the nonsaturable elimination component becomes dominant and controls the new half-life, with negligible contribution from the saturable component. The effect of drug concentrations on the half-life of drugs that are cleared by nonsaturable, saturable, and combined saturable and nonsaturable pathways is shown in Figure 16.4.

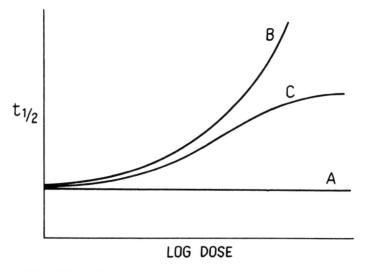

Figure 16.4. Changes in apparent elimination half-life with increasing dose for drugs that are cleared from the body by A, nonsaturable; B, saturable; and C, parallel saturable and nonsaturable pathways.

An important consequence of the increase in apparent drug half-life with increasing drug concentrations is increased and prolonged drug accumulation with repeated dosing. Levy and Tsuchiya (9) showed that a twofold increase in salicylate dosage from 0.5 to 1 g every 8 h could result in a more than sixfold increase in steady-state salicylate levels. An increase in the time to reach steady state from 2 to 7 days also occurs.

Area Under the Drug Concentration Curve. As long as a drug obeys linear kinetics, and provided the kinetics are dose-independent, the AUC will be directly proportional to the available dose. This relationship is shown in Equation 16.20 for the one-compartment model.

$$AUC^{0 \to \infty} = D/Vk_{el} \tag{16.20}$$

For drugs that obey saturable kinetics, however, this relationship may not be the case. The AUC after intravenous injection of a drug that is eliminated by a single saturable pathway is given by

$$AUC^{0 \to \infty} - (C_o/V_m)[(C_o/2) + K_m] \tag{16.21}$$

When the initial drug level, C_o, is much less than K_m, Equation 16.21 reduces to Equation 16.22.

$$AUC^{0 \to \infty} = (C_o K_m/V_m) = (D \cdot K_m)/(V \cdot V_m) = D/(V \cdot k) \tag{16.22}$$

In this situation, the AUC is again directly proportional to the dose, just as in the first-order elimination case. However, if C_o is much greater than K_m, then Equation 16.21 becomes

$$AUC^{0 \to \infty} = C_o^2/2V_m = D^2/(2 \cdot V^2 \cdot V_m) \tag{16.23}$$

Quite a different situation is obtained in this equation because the AUC is proportional to the square of the dose and inversely proportional to the square of the distribution volume. However, the distribution volume should remain constant and should not influence drug levels from different doses.

Thus, the more drug concentrations lie within the saturable range, the greater the tendency for AUC values to increase disproportionately with increasing dose. The example represented by Equation 16.23 is based on simple kinetics associated with intravenous dosing and the one-compartment kinetic model. However, the problem of disproportionate increases in AUC values with small dose increments is independent of dosage route and the kinetic model.

First-Pass Metabolism. Most drugs are metabolized predominantly in the liver, which is the site where saturation of metabolism is most likely to occur. Because saturation occurs at high drug concentrations, the time saturation is most likely to occur is during drug absorption via the splanchnic circulation and the portal vein. Drug concentrations are generally much higher at this time than after they have entered the general circulation (i.e., during the first pass through the liver). This high drug concentration can lead to saturation of drug-metabolizing enzymes during absorption and hence greater bioavailability of unchanged drug. Because saturation occurs at high drug concentrations, a rapidly absorbed drug is likely to undergo less first-pass metabolism than a more slowly absorbed drug. This situation is a potentially serious problem for sustained-release dosage forms. If a drug undergoes saturable metabolism, then the slower the release and hence the lower the drug concentrations in the splanchnic circulation, the greater the opportunity for first-pass metabolism. Therefore, accurate determination of the relative bioavailability of slow release dosage forms compared to conventional dosage forms or oral solutions is important.

An interesting example of possible saturation of hepatic metabolizing enzymes during the first pass is provided by the anticancer compound 5-fluorouracil. This drug is extensively metabolized in the body and has a very short biological half-life of about 10 min. With such a short half-life, the drug would be expected to be extensively metabolized during the first pass after oral dosing and result in less than 5% bioavailability. In fact, 5-fluorouracil is absorbed reasonably well after oral doses, and the AUC from equivalent oral doses is approximately 30% of that after intravenous injection. So it appears (and remains to be proven) that the high oral dose of approximately 1 g of 5-fluorouracil is capable of saturating the hepatic enzymes during the first pass, resulting in more efficient absorption of unchanged drug than would be predicted.

Summary

1. Most drugs are eliminated from the body by mechanisms that are potentially saturable. True first-order, nonsaturable elimination occurs only with drugs that are excreted in urine via passive glomerular filtration.

2. Some drugs exhibit saturable elimination at therapeutic blood concentrations.

3. A drug that is cleared by zero-order or Michaelis–Menten-type kinetics does not exhibit a characteristic, constant elimination half-life. The apparent half-life changes continuously with drug concentration in plasma.

4. Saturable first-pass metabolism may lead to increased absorption efficiency of drug from a rapid-release oral formulation compared with a slow-release oral formulation.

5. Saturable elimination may introduce bias into systemic availability estimates of drug from fast- and slow- release formulations and from large versus small oral doses.

Literature Cited

1. Jusko, W. J.; Levy, G. *J. Pharm. Sci.*, **1970**, *59*, 765–772.
2. Lundquist, F.; Wolthers, H. *Acta Pharmacol. Toxicol.*, **1958**, *14*, 265–289.
3. Winek, C. L. *Trial*, **1983**, *19*, 38.
4. Welling, P. G.; Lyons, L. L.; Elliot, R.; Amidon, G. L. *J. Clin. Pharmacol.*, **1977**, *17*, 199–206.
5. Arnold, K.; Gerber, N. *Clin. Pharmacol. Ther.*, **1970**, *11*, 121–134.
6. Dayton, P. G.; Cucinell, C. A.; Weiss, M.; Perell, J. M. *J. Pharmacol. Exp. Ther.*, **1967**, *158*, 305–316.
7. Levy, G. *J. Pharm. Sci.*, **1965**, *54*, 959–967.
8. Selen, A.; Amidon, G. L.; Welling, P. G. *J. Pharm. Sci.*, **1982**, *71*, 1238–1241.
9. Levy, G.; Tsuchiya, T. *New Engl. J. Med.*, **1972**, *287*, 430–432.
10. Levy, G.; Tsuchiya, T.; Amsel, L. P. *Clin. Pharmacol. Ther.*, **1972**, *13*, 258–268.
11. Wagner, J. G.; *Fundamentals of Clinical Pharmacokinetics*; Drug Intelligence Publications: Hamilton, IL, 1975, pp 247–284.

Problems

1. A drug that undergoes saturable elimination has a V_m of 10 μg/mL · h and a K_m of 20 μg/mL. What are (i) the apparent first-order elimination rate constant and (ii) the apparent biological half-life of the drug when circulating drug levels are below the saturation range?

2. Following bolus intravenous injection of a drug that obeys one-compartment kinetics and exhibits saturable elimination, the observed maximum drug concentration in plasma obtained immediately after dosing was 8 μg/mL. The drug concentration in plasma obtained by extrapolating the terminal log-linear portion of the drug concentration curve back to zero time was 13.5 μg/mL, and the apparent half-life from the log-linear elimination phase was 1.5 h. Calculate V_m and K_m from these data.

3. A person who weighs 150 lb will attain a blood alcohol concentration (BAC) of approximately 0.025 percent upon complete absorption of 12 oz of beer (4% ethanol, 8 proof) or 1 oz of 100-proof (50% ethanol) liquor. During the zero-order elimination range, the average rate of ethanol elimination from the blood is 0.018%/h.

   A 150-lb person started drinking at 6:00 p.m. and continued until 10:00 p.m. During that time the person drank six 12-oz bottles of beer. What was the person's BAC at 11:00 p.m.?

4. How many ounces of 100-proof (50% ethanol) liquor would a 150-lb person have to drink between 6:00 and 10:00 p.m. to have a blood alcohol content of 0.1 mg% at 11:00 p.m.?

5. A single 100-mg oral dose tablet of a drug that is eliminated by a single saturable pathway yielded a peak plasma drug concentration of 17 μg/mL approximately 2 h postdose. Reformulation into a fast-release suspension resulted in a peak plasma level of 25 μg/

mL from the same dose size, occurring at 0.5 h. Calculate (i) the approximate increase in AUC that results from the fast-release suspension compared to the slower release tablet formulation, and (ii) to what level the fast-release dosage would have to be reduced to yield the same AUC as the slower release formulation. K_m is 0.5 μg/mL.

Appendix I—Answers to Problems

Chapter 4   1. 0.67 or 67%
                2. 50%

Chapter 7   1. 12 L
                2. 25 L
                3. $C_F = 1.45\ \mu g/mL$, $C_B = 13.05\ \mu g/mL$, $C_T = 14.5\ \mu g/ml$, $A_F = 60.9$ mg (%), $V_{app} = 6.9$ L
                4. $C_F = 0.44\ \mu g/mL$, $C_B = 3.96\ \mu g/mL$, $C_T = 4.4\ \mu g/mL$, $A_F = 18.5$ mg (%), $V_{app} = 22.7$ L
                5. $C_F = 0.49\ \mu g/mL$, $C_B = 0.74\ \mu g/mL$, $C_T = 1.23\ \mu g/mL$, $A_F = 20.6$ mg (%), $V_{app} = 81.3$ L

Chapter 9   1. 300 mL/min
                2. 600 mL/min
                3. 0.81 h
                4. No

Chapter 10   1. Both the same
                2. 116 mL/min
                3. 0.25
                4. 49.4 L
                5. (i) 6.93 h, (ii) $0.1\ h^{-1}$, (iii) 22.4 L, (iv) 37.3 mL/min
                6. (i) $175.3\ \mu g \cdot h/mL$, (ii) $202.3\ \mu g \cdot h/mL$

7. (i) 5.0 h, (ii) 28 mL/min, (iii) 28 mL/min,
   (iv) 20.8 µg/mL, 18.1 µg/mL, (v) 148.8 µg · h/mL
8. (i) 39 µg/mL, (ii) 19.4 h, 29.9 h
9. (i) 13 µg/mL, (ii) 6.48 h, 9.96 h
10. k_0 = 1.5 mg/min, No
11. At 1 h, C = 24.6 µg/mL
    At 10 h, C = 0.38 µg/mL
12. 194.8 ≃ 195 mg

Chapter 11   1. (i) 577.2 µg · h/mL, (ii) 30.7 µg/mL, (iii) 1.43 h
2. (i) 865.8 µg · h/mL, (ii) 31.4 µg/mL, (iii) 1.57 h
3. 0.89
4. (i) 0.2 h^{-1}, (ii) 55.6 mg
5. (i) 0.2 h^{-1}, (ii) 3.5 h, (iii) 1.5 h^{-1}, (iv) 0.46 h,
   (v) 19.1 L, (vi) 63 mL/min
6. (i) 0.2 h^{-1}, (ii) 0.15 h^{-1}, (iii) 0.05 h^{-1}
7. 47.75 mL/min

Chapter 12   1. (i) 2.38 µg/mL, (ii) 4.76 µg/mL, (iii) 2.38 µg/mL,
   (iv) 3.43 µg/mL
2. (i) 9.63 µg/mL, (ii) 6.06 µg/mL, (iii) 7.69 µg/mL
3. (i) 40.2 µg/mL, (ii) 4.3 doses, (iii) 34.6 ≃ 36 h
4. (i) 63.3 µg/mL, (ii) 8.6 doses, (iii) 34.6 ≃ 36 h
5. (i) 82 µg/mL, (ii) 10.8 ≃ 11 doses, (iii) 86.4 h
6. 40 mg
7. 20 h
8. 200 mg
9. (i) 3.2 h, (ii) 2.18 h

Chapter 13   1. (i) 0.45 h^{-1}, (ii) 0.15 h^{-1}, (iii) 0.2 h^{-1}
2. (i) 0.2 h^{-1}, (ii) 0.1 h^{-1}, (iii) 1.5 h^{-1}
3. 0.23 h^{-1}
4. 4 h
5. 6 h

Chapter 14   1. (i) 15 L, (ii) 18.3 L, (iii) 12.5 L, (iv) 25 mL/min,
   (v) 13.8 mL/min
2. 2.8 h
3. 212 mL/min
4. 1.2 h
5. Triphasic
6. 2.17 h
7. 394.5 µg · h/mL
8. 3.38 mL/min
9. (i) 2.54 mL/min, (ii) 0.85 mL/min

Chapter 15   1. (i) 0.38, (ii) 456 mL/min
             2. 1
             3. 6 μg/mL
             4. 1.8 μg/mL
             5. (i) 336 mL/min, (ii) 7.5 μg/mL, (iii) 13.4 μg/mL

Chapter 16   1. (i) 0.5 h^{-1}, (ii) 1.39 h
             2. (i) 15.3 μg/mL, (ii) 7.06 μg · h/mL
             3. 0.06 mg %
             4. 7.6 oz
             5. (i) 2.2-fold, (ii) 46-mg dose.

Appendix II—Nomenclature

A	(1) Amount of drug in the body (numerical subscript indicates compartment); (2) intercept of α slope of blood level curve at $t = 0$ in two-compartment model
AAG	α_1-Acid glycoprotein
A_0	Amount of drug in the body at zero time
A_F	Amount of free drug in the body
A_T	Amount of total drug in the body
A_u	Cumulative urinary recovery of unchanged drug
A_u^∞	Total urinary recovery of unchanged drug
$A_{n(\max)}$	Maximum amount of drug in the body after n doses
$A_{n(\min)}$	Minimum amount of drug in the body after n doses
$A_{n(t)}$	Amount of drug in the body at any time during a dosage interval after n doses
A_{ss}	Amount of drug in the body at steady state during zero-order input
$A_{1(2)}$	Amount of drug in first or second compartment of the two-compartment model
$\text{AUC}^{0 \to t}$	Area under drug concentration curve from zero to time t
$\text{AUC}^{0 \to \infty}$	Area under drug concentration curve from zero to infinite time
$\text{AUC}^{0 \to \tau}$	Area under drug concentration curve during a multiple dosage interval, at steady state
$\text{AUMC}^{0 \to \infty}$	Area under the moment curve from zero to infinite time
α	Fast composite rate constant for the two-compartment open model
B	Intercept of β slope of blood level curve at $t = 0$ in two-compartment model
β	(1) Slow composite rate constant for the two-compartment open model; (2) fraction of drug bound in plasma

C	Drug concentration (subscript indicates fluid, tissue, or compartment, bound or unbound)
C'	Intercept of k_a slope of drug plasma concentration curve at $t = 0$ in two-compartment model
C_i	Drug concentration in afferent blood
C_o	Concentration of drug in efferent blood
C_0	Initial drug concentration
C_{max}	Peak or maximum drug concentration
$C_{n(max)}$	Maximum concentration of drug after n doses
$C_{n(min)}$	Minimum concentration of drug after n doses
$C_{n(t)}$	Concentration of drug at any time during a dosing interval after n doses
$C_{\infty(max)}$	Maximum drug concentration after repeated doses, at steady state
$C_{\infty(min)}$	Minimum drug concentration after repeated doses, at steady state
$C_{\infty(t)}$	Concentration of drug at any time during a dosing interval, at steady state.
$\overline{C}_{\infty}$	Average drug concentration during a repeated dose interval, at steady state
C_{ss}	Drug concentration at steady state during zero-order drug input
C_t	Drug concentration at sampling time t after a single dose
Cl_{cr}	Creatinine clearance
Cl_T	Drug clearance by particular tissue T
Cl_p	Plasma clearance
Cl_r	Renal clearance
ΔC	Change in drug concentration during time interval Δt
D	Dose
E_H	Hepatic extraction ratio
E	Extraction ratio of any organ
ESR	Erythrocyte sedimentation rate
ϵ	(1) Ratio of bound to free drug in extravascular fluids; (2) the ratio $\tau:t_{1/2}$ during repeated drug doses
F	Fraction of administered dose that is available to the systemic circulation
f	Fraction of drug that is cleared unchanged in urine
f'	Fraction of drug that is cleared as a metabolite
f_T	Free drug fraction in tissue T
γ	Ratio of bound to free drug in plasma
K	Drug–protein equilibrium dissociation constant
K_m	Michaelis constant
K_p	Equilibrium distribution ratio
k	First-order rate constant
k_a	First-order rate constant for appearance of drug into the systemic circulation
k_{ab}	Intrinsic first-order rate constant for drug absorption

k_d	First-order rate constant for drug degradation at the absorption site
k_e	First-order rate constant for urinary excretion of unchanged drug
k_{el}	First-order rate constant for drug elimination by all routes
k_m	First-order rate constant for drug metabolism
k_{me}	First-order rate constant for urinary excretion of a metabolite
k_n	First-order elimination rate constant for a drug under condition of normal renal function
k_{nr}	First-order rate constant for drug elimination by nonrenal mechanisms
k_0	Zero-order rate constant for drug absorption
k_u	First-order elimination rate constant for a drug under condition of uremia
k_{12}	First-order rate constant for transfer of drug from the first compartment to the second compartment of the two-compartment open model
k_{21}	First-order rate constant for transfer of drug from the second compartment to the first compartment of the two-compartment open model
λ	A first-order rate constant
M	Amount of metabolite in the body
M_u	Cumulative urinary recovery of metabolite
M_u^∞	Total urinary recovery of metabolite
n	Number of binding sites per protein molecule
P	Quantity of drug in plasma compartment
$[P]$	Protein concentration
$[P_f]$	Concentration of free receptors on protein
$[P_fC]$	Concentration of combined receptors
Q	Blood flow rate (subscript indicates to a particular organ)
R	(1) Residual obtained by drug level curve-stripping; (2) accumulation factor during repeated drug dose; (3) partition coefficient for drug disposition into organ (subscript) at equilibrium
R_T	Partition coefficient of total drug between tissue T and blood, at equilibrium
r	Number of moles of drug bound to a mole of protein
T	(1) Duration of zero-order drug input; (2) quantity of drug in tissue compartment
t	Time elapsed since a single drug dose
t_0	Lag time. The time interval between drug administration and the first appearance of measurable drug in the circulation
t'	Time elapsed since end of zero-order drug release
$t_{1/2}$	Drug elimination half-life
$t_{1/2n}$	Drug elimination half-life under condition of normal renal function
$t_{1/2u}$	Drug elimination half-life under condition of uremia

T_{max}	Time of peak or maximum drug concentration
$T_{\infty(max)}$	Time of maximum drug concentration during repeated doses, at steady state
τ	Dosage interval
U	Concentration of drug in urine
V	Volume (subscript indicates fluid, tissue, or compartment)
V'	Urine flow rate
V_{app}	Apparent drug body distribution volume
V_{dss}	Overall distribution volume of a drug that obeys two-compartment model kinetics
$V_{d(extrap)}$	Overall distribution volume of a drug that obeys two-compartment model kinetics, calculated by extrapolation method
$V_{d(area)}$, $V_d\beta$	Overall distribution volume of a drug that obeys two-compartment model kinetics, calculated by area method
V_m, V_{max}	Maximum rate of elimination in a saturable system
X	Amount of drug remaining to be absorbed

GLOSSARY

active transport membrane transport that uses cellular energy for drug movement, with or against a concentration gradient.

amorphic forms polymorphs that have no crystal structure.

blood–brain barrier defense structure that minimizes access of water-soluble substances to the brain.

catenary chain kinetics sequence of kinetic steps in the form A→B→C.

diffusion rate-limited dependent on the rate at which drug molecules can diffuse across the membrane.

enteral administration drug administration via the GI tract.

enterohepatic circulation continuous recirculation of substance between liver and intestine by means of the bile.

intact nephron hypothesis hypothesis stating that the diseased kidney is considered to comprise variable ratios of normal nephrons and nephrons that are essentially nonfunctional due to the pathological condition.

intravenous administration direct administration of drug into the venous circulation by means of syringe or intravenous line.

microsomes liver fraction, obtained from sequential cenrifugation of liver homogenate, associated with drug metabolism.

parenteral administration drug administration via any route other than the GI tract.

passive transfer mechanism of membrane transport that depends on the concentration gradient of substance across the membrane.

passive-facilitated diffusion membrane crossing driven by a concentration gradient.

perfusion rate-limited dependent on how fast a particular tissue is perfused by blood.

plasma clear supernate recovered after red blood cells have been precipitated, obtained from a blood sample in the presence of an anticoagulant.

plasma clearance   volume of plasma cleared of drug per unit time as a result of all elimination pathways.

plasma half-life   time taken for drug concentration in plasma to be reduced by one-half.

polymorphs   compounds that can form crystals with different molecular arrangements.

renal clearance   volume of plasma cleared of drug per unit time as a result of urinary excretion.

serum   clear supernate recovered after red cells have been allowed to clot, obtained from a blood sample in the absence of an anticoagulant.

solvates   crystals that incorporate one or more solvent molecules during preparation.

solvation   incorporation of one or more solvent molecules into the crystalline structure of a substance.

systemically acting drugs   drugs that must enter the systemic circulation to exert their therapeutic effect.

thekes   Greek word meaning sheath or box; derivation of intrathecal administration.

INDEX

INDEX

O

Ocular drug administration, 165
One-compartment open model
  bolus intravenous injection, 5*f*
  concentration versus time profile, 168*f*
  first-order absorption and elimination,
    163, 164*f*, 257*s*
  logarithm of drug concentration versus
    time, 166*f*
  Michaelis constants, 262*f*
  obtaining parameters from a blood-level
    profile, 166–171
  routes of elimination, 140, 258*s*
  use, 140
  zero-order absorption and first-order
    elimination, 141*s*, 152–159
Oral bioavailability, best dosage form, 46
Oral dosage forms, zero-order, 158
Organ, drug elimination rate, 244
Organ clearance, 243–245
Organ extraction ratio
  definition, 244
  values for eliminating organs, 244–245
Oxidations
  benzyl alcohol, 109*s*
  ethanol, 109*s*
Oxidative deamination, amphetamine, 108*s*
Oxidative reactions, biological half-life
  influenced, 110

P

Parenteral administration, 2, 7–19
Particle size
  drug absorption effect, 43
  reduction, 43
Partition coefficient, distribution of drug
  from blood to tissue, 248
Passive facilitated diffusion, 24–25
Passive transfer, membrane crossing, 23–24
Penicillamine, effect of ferrous sulfate and
  antacid mixtures, 71
Penicillin
  effect of food on absorption, 70
  loading dose required to reach steady
    state, 195
  plasma levels in fasting subjects, 40
Penicillin G benzathine, sustained increase,
  9
Penicillin G procaine, sustained increase, 9
Pentothal, apparent distribution volume,
  79
Percutaneous absorption, description, 10,
  13
Perfusion rate limited, definition, 80
  definition, 80
  transport examples, 82
  See also Blood flow rate-limited transport
Peritonitis, disadvantage of self-
  administered CAPD, 17–18
pH, strong base and weak acid solution,
  40–41
Pharmacokinetic compartment, use,
  139–140

Pharmacokinetics
  controlled release, 56
  definition, 3–4
  mathematics, 161–268
  modeling approaches, 4–6
Pharmacological activity
  loss, 105
  organs, 245
Pharmacology, definition, 3
Phase I oxidation reactions, 107–109*f*
Phase I reduction reactions, 110–111*f*
Phenobarbital
  formation, 106
  oral doses, 164
  rate constant determination, 170
Phenylbutazone, plasma half-life, 117
Phenytoin, protein binding, 87–88
Physiological models, 241–253
  advantages, 242
  anticancer compounds, 253
  basic unit, 5*f*
  blood, muscle, and kidney, 247*s*
  choice of organs included, 245–251
  complications, 242
  derivation of mathematical expressions,
    247
  description, 4–5, 241–243
  digoxin disposition in the rat, 6*f*
  disadvantages, 242–243
  drugs acting on the CNS, 253
  equations for complex models, 249
  experimental considerations, 252–254
  organ capable of drug elimination, 243*s*
  membrane-limited transport expressions,
    252
Planimetry, used to calculate AUC, 145
Plasma
  AUC, 192*f*
  concentration of free drug, 88
  definition, 78
  drug concentrations in whole blood,
    extracellular, and intracellular water,
    78
  drug loss model for urinary excretion
    and metabolism, 126*f*
  maximum drug concentration, 191
  ratio of drug quantity to that in tissue,
    226–227
  terminal linear portion of the metabolite
    profile, 205
Plasma clearance
  definition, 123
  determination, 125–126
  differentiated from renal clearance,
    125
  equation, 143
  obtained from AUC, 144
  obtained from multiple-dose data,
    191–192
  two-compartment model, 222, 224
Plasma half-life
  definition, 127
  relationship to drug distribution volume,
    128
Plasma proteins, drug binding, 78–79,
  82–88, 91, 94

Editing and indexing by Keith B. Belton
Production by Joan C. Cook
Jacket design by Pamela Lewis
Managing Editor: Janet S. Dodd

Typeset by Techna Type, Inc., York, PA, and
Hot Type Ltd., Washington, DC
Printed and bound by Maple Press Company, York, PA